THE SUNSHINE PRINCIPLE

A RADICALLY SIMPLE GUIDE TO NATURAL CATHOLIC HEALING

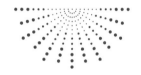

MELODY LYONS

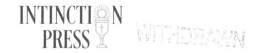

INTINCTION PRESS

COPYRIGHT

This book contains the opinions and ideas of its author. It is solely for informational and educational purposes and should not be regarded as a substitute for professional medical advice or treatment. The nature of your health needs is complex and unique. Therefore, you should consult a health professional before you begin any exercise, nutrition, or supplementation program or if you have questions about your health. Neither the author nor the publisher shall be liable or responsible for any loss or damage allegedly arising from any information or suggestion in this book.

The Sunshine Principle: A Radically Simple Guide to Natural Catholic Healing/Melody Lyons — 1st ed.

ISBN: 978-1-953644-00-8

To my husband, Christopher.
You carry me in sickness and in health as though I am light as a feather.

CONTENTS

INTRODUCTION

The Sunshine Principle is simply this: that the greatest potential for healing occurs when we align our behaviors with God's design.

The message of the Sunshine Principle is expressed repeatedly in the Church's moral teachings, Sacred Scripture, and Sacred Tradition. Once the gimmicks, verbiage, and misunderstandings related to natural wellness are stripped away, we are left with a simple formula based on God's design for creation and His great love for us.

Every detail of daily living—from what we eat to how we pray—is illuminated by this principle, making healing possible, accessible, and joyful! My own story is a testimony to the truth of God's love and attentiveness through His natural gifts. Like Elijah's travels through the wilderness in 1 Kings 19, it has been a tale of what seems miraculous—not by a suspension of God's law but *through* God's law. And the amazing truth is that the resources for natural healing are available to you as well!

Elijah was exhausted, afraid, alone. Perhaps you are also very near the end of your emotional and mental limitations. This book is for you. It is a bridge for the seeker who wants to explore alternatives to pharmaceuticals without falling into the errors of New Age earth- or body-worship. After Elijah rested, the angel commanded him to get up and eat so that he might be strong for the journey. In a similar way, this book considers a simple plan to help gently restore an individual, familial, and cultural vision that God intended for His beloved people.

The natural world belongs to God. He is Master of all creation, including all life and its activity. Non-believers may make use of a plant or move their bodies in a secular or profane way, but this does not make them master over those things. Because it is the revealed truth of God, Catholicism recognizes the beautiful integration of mind, body, and soul in a way that surpasses all other belief systems. This recognition of the gifts inherent in the created world flows quite naturally from our relationship with Our Father, the giver of all that is good.

My desire is to help restore and develop a culture of intuitive health care and healing, which flows from the Gospel and is guided by the principle of subsidiarity. This is not to disregard the role of reason in discerning and judging what is good and true—reason is essential. Rather, it recognizes, as St. Thomas points out, that "in God, there is a sure judgement of truth...by simple intuition." (ST II-II, q. 9, a. 2)

The enemies of God want us sick, depressed, anxious, drugged, confused, oppressed, and defeated. I will not comply. I reject those obstacles which dull the senses and make the body ill or more inclined to despair. I will fight for joy, strength, hope, and clarity—God created this body to serve Him. Serviam!

Our Lady, Star of the Sea...

St. Hildegard of Bingen...

St. Dominic de Guzman...

Ora Pro Nobis.

THE SUNSHINE PRINCIPLE

God has arranged everything in the universe in consideration of everything else. — St. Hildegard of Bingen

---

*M*y story of healing is a testimony of gratitude and praise and, like the deaf-mute of the Scriptures, I cannot stay silent. Many would consider my healing nothing short of miraculous. During a miracle, the normal laws of science are suspended. On the other hand, mine is a personal history of truly amazing transformation, not by a suspension of God's laws but *through* God's laws. This sort of healing is accessible to the multitude of people who are hurting and begging for help, but who habitually (and perhaps obliviously) reject the means which God has already provided.

For most of my life, I viewed the notion of health through the blurry lens of modern culture instead of the Church's expansive and telescopic vision of Salvation History. When I heard the term "natural healing," I reflexively thought of aging hippies smoking weed and fondling crystals instead of the glorious narrative of creation! I didn't grasp the inadequacy of my understanding until the ingenuity of mankind failed me during a health crisis and I was able to find healing only through natural options.

I wrote this book as an act of praise and thanksgiving. My primary goal is to help others also find healing in God's natural design. I also hope to bridge the growing gap between modern American culture and the truth expressed in God's creation. Our post-Christian culture has largely lost sight of the latter and, in so doing, has lost an essential connection with God Himself. In an age when God is often reported dead, we have tried to replace faith with a foolish anthropogenic view of creation. Rejecting God as the Creator and Author of life, this view also dismisses His created, natural world as the primary source of healing. This defective view claims: if *we* didn't make it or perfect it, then it must be inferior.

No thanks ... I'm just not into that natural stuff. We're all going to die anyway! Give me a soda and ibuprofen and I'll give thanks to God for the gift of technology.

Of course, it would be lunacy to reject the truly beneficial medical and technological advancements of our time! However, true healing for the Christian (indeed, for anyone) requires connecting with God through the created world and rising above a shallow relationship with our surroundings It also demands that we take a second analytical look at the last 50-100 years of medical history, and that we remain open to reconsidering some of the wisdom gained prior to— and rejected during—this present age. Because so much knowledge of and reverence for God's creation has been lost, some are left with the bizarre inclination to say, "I just don't believe all that natural stuff. It might interfere with my statins." Instead, they should be asking, "What is the most direct and effective method of lowering my cholesterol, and in harmony with God's design for my body?"

The answer is obvious—and I don't know a physician who will

disagree—that it is not usually nature which is lacking, but our failure to honor the most fundamental needs of the body. We live and eat poorly, and stubbornly refuse to change our habits. This reveals either a fundamental lack of trust in the God of Genesis who missed nothing in providing for our well-being, or perhaps a carefully nurtured indolence grown accustomed to convenience-food wrapped in cellophane. Whatever the reasons, it seems that we often don't really want to do it His way.

In one small way at least, I am like the Apostle Paul: I don't want you to follow me, but Him. The purpose of this book is to point you that way. My objective is not to convince you to throw away your statins or Beta-blockers (unless you don't want and no longer need them) but to help you grow closer to God in every area of your life.

This premise condenses into one simple principle inspired by natural law, the teachings of the Church, and the writings of St. Hildegard of Bingen.

That principle—which I call the Sunshine Principle—is that **God has arranged everything in the universe in consideration of everything else, and the greatest potential for healing occurs when we align our behaviors with God's natural, biological, and spiritual laws.**

This truth is so obvious in every aspect of life and faith that it stands like the sun—unfailing, necessary, and powerful, but so often taken for granted. Like grown-ups who cannot return to Narnia, we have long since ceased to be awed. We have forgotten that it was made for us; that all of creation was designed for our benefit. This book is not a complicated re-presentation of the truth, but merely a gentle and joyful reminder. God has set all things in motion in consideration of us ... his beloved.

For those who have never before seriously considered the idea of natural health care, it is also an introduction to the Church's wisdom in this area and a basic guide to living more closely united to God's glorious design.

My hope is that this book will be a small bridge between our cultural misunderstanding of the natural world and God's plan for our healing. The hijacking of the holy naturalist and Doctor of the Church, Saint Hildegard of Bingen, by those who do not love Christ is a perfect example of how this confusion can occur.

Many involved in New Age, eco-feminism, and pagan worship have purposefully fostered a misunderstanding of St. Hildegard (as they do to so much of God's natural order). But they have been forced to remake her in their own image to explain away her fervent obedience. They miss the point that connecting and yielding to God's order ultimately brings the greatest freedom. She was a spirited, bold, prolific, artistic, preaching polymath, and yet still submissive to the laws of Christ, the teachings of the Church, and the Rule of Saint Benedict.

St. Hildegard is an enigma to many Catholics who are not accustomed to speaking with passion and fire about God and His treasures made manifest in humanity. We want a neat pill and she offers us a messy poultice. We want a snappy hymn and she composes a lengthy mystical piece. We don't want to rock the boat and she publicly admonishes priests and bishops against their corruption. We think of her (incorrectly) as a habited hippie and we don't know how to integrate who *we* are with her expression of adamant faith.

The wonderful truth is that the very dynamic cultivation of the life of Christ in the soul of St. Hildegard during her early life brought forth the explosion of creativity later. It was not only the natural world which inspired Hildegard's joy, but the Creator Himself to Whom she oriented all of her work and love. Those who focus their adoration on the creation seem to forget the Creator. Like the poor pagans surrounding Abram in Haran, they have busied themselves about worshipping the sunshine instead of receiving it. It is but one example of the pitfalls of the modern secular subculture of "natural healing" which I hope to correct in these pages.

I once participated in a peg doll swap with local Catholic women and decided to paint St. Hildegard, knowing that my contribution might be misunderstood by other attendees. One woman finally asked: "So why *did* you choose Hildegard?" From the tone of her voice, I knew she was skeptical of my motives. I quickly reassured her that no, I'm not a militant anti-patriarchal feminist…I'm just attempting to bring Hildegard into her rightful place with all the other Church-loving saints (in peg form, of course.)

I appreciated both her query and her wariness. In the battle to conform our souls to Christ, we must be radically committed to love. This means guarding our hearts against the multitude of attacks against the Faith, both ancient and modern. We must also be intellectually engaged so that we will not be robbed of our heritage with a persuasive (but false) narrative. We are called to be protective of the natural world and be proactive in our efforts to restore its place in our lives.

Prior to her 42nd year, St. Hildegard lived her life quietly and under the rule of her order. During that time, it might be said that she grew in wisdom, age, and grace. Certainly, she developed the virtue, discipline, passionate love, and obedience which would pour forth from her much more publicly in mid-life and beyond.

I am typing out these words during my own (much less impressive) 42nd year, praying for renewal in the Church. I am also praying that we will learn to embrace faithful dynamic adherence to the laws of Christ, which are expressed through every jot and tittle of creation.

The Lord by wisdom founded the earth; by understanding he established the heavens; by his knowledge the deeps broke forth, and the clouds drop down the dew. Proverbs 3:19-20

I want to begin this book with a particular word of hope for those of you reading in the midst of a health crisis:

The greatest portion of St. Hildegard's known work was done after she fell ill, in the midst of continuous health struggles, and when she was past mid-life.

And you?

Your work is not done.

Your fire is not extinguished.

Be open to the idea that God's greatest work through you will pour forth irrespective of whether or not you feel equipped for it. Be open to healing in ways you never expected.

2

RISE AND EAT!

Which is easier, to say, 'Your sins are forgiven,' or to say, 'Rise and walk'? — Matthew 9:5

I resolved to write this book in the midst of a brutally difficult Spring morning. I sat at my desk with my head in my arms, bawling like a baby. It had been a tough week. My autoimmune disease had flared and I was looking for a little relief by reading my favorite internet health gurus. With a news feed full of natural wellness gold, I had been earnestly taking notes for fifteen minutes. And then...I just fell apart.

I cried until my nose ran. I was completely overwhelmed. What I really needed was a good long nap, a professional back rub, a personal chef, a date with my husband, and a cure for lupus! I would have settled for the nap. Instead, my mind was overloaded by digital images of infrared saunas, squatty potties, and 1001 ways to use bone broth. I wasn't opposed to those things necessarily but, on that particular day,

I just needed one helpful thing. And I didn't even know which one it was.

Too tired to care and too upset to continue, I closed my laptop, cried it out for a bit, and then I laid down on my bed in spite of the fact that it was only noon. It turns out that a nap truly was the one thing I needed. Sometimes the simplest path to healing is finding one small thing and just beginning. The littlest way.

As I awoke from this brief respite and pondered this tiny midday gift, my mind naturally turned to St. Therese of Lisieux—to her simple way of expressing loving in the midst of suffering. I begged her to accompany me and teach me acceptance and courage, and I was consoled. In what seemed like a direct answer to that prayer, I was led to the Biblical story of the account of Elijah fleeing from Jezebel into the wilderness (1 Kings 19):

But he himself went a day's journey into the wilderness, and came and sat down under a broom tree; and he asked that he might die, saying, "It is enough; now, O Lord, take away my life; for I am no better than my fathers.

So far, this was feeling like my travels. Elijah and me...desperate, tired...done. It is enough!

And he lay down and slept under a broom tree; and behold, an angel touched him, and said to him, "Arise and eat." And he looked, and behold, there was at his head a cake baked on hot stones and a jar of water. And he ate and drank, and lay down again. And the angel of the Lord came again a second time, and touched him, and said, "Arise and eat, else the journey will be too great for you." And he arose, and ate and drank, and went in the strength of that food forty days and forty nights to Horeb the mount of God.

I was amazed and overwhelmed. Through that passage, I heard the Lord speak into my fear, my pain, and my hopelessness:

GET UP AND EAT.

Rising up, I willed myself to take my supplements and made a quick and nourishing lunch. I did a couple other things that mothers must do (changed a diaper, read a book to a little one, and briefly debated with a teenager), and then sat down to type out some thoughts about this complicated journey of chronic illness and my search for hope. The exercise turned out to be cathartic. The lasting result is this legacy for my children and anyone else who needs just one small inspiration to be able to rise.

WHERE DO YOU NEED HEALING?

We are all seeking healing in some area of our lives. It is, without a doubt, the birthright of our fallen nature. I am eager to share with you everything that I have learned about how to heal. But I also want to honor your pace and guard the door for you while you take that badly needed nap. I hope to be your sister on the journey, who loves you enough to share what is good and offer a word of encouragement.

The Sunshine Principle cuts through the confusion because it helps us sift through the distractions and just do the one thing in the moment that brings us closer to healing.

The angel of the Lord could have taken Elijah for a miraculous flight across the wilderness. God could have suspended his natural need for food, sleep, and water. But He didn't. Rather, He chose the normal physical means of food and sleep to refresh Elijah and to sustain Him on a difficult journey. Although the appearance of the cake and water was miraculous, the Scriptures make clear that the cake was "baked on hot stones" and that Elijah needed to physically eat it in order to complete his travels. What a perfect reminder that these simple healing actions are not an inconvenient obstacle, but the *primary* means by which we are to be restored!

In a similar act of benevolence, God sent the angel Raphael to heal Tobit of his blindness by applying fish gall to his eyes. Honestly, my first thought as an American suburbanite who grew up with packaged foods and standardized medicine was: *Yuck. Why did God choose the gall of a fish?* Was it just some random slimy vehicle for supernatural blessing? Or did God choose the fish gall because he had designed the chemistry of that gall to be exactly suited to Tobit's biological need? Either way, it is the divine healing power of God, expressed through the natural order. I am again reminded of Saint Hildegard who observed that God's presence in the design of His creation is altogether miraculous.

I have learned through my experience of illness that, even while I beg God to instantly heal me, I should accept that the answer to my prayer will likely come from sustained study and effort. Whenever I experience an overwhelming day and my body just doesn't seem to respond to my diligent application of time and resources, I return to the essentials. One meal at a time. One supplement at a time. One walk, nap, prayer, song at a time. There is no magic pill, but I am living proof that there is hope.

After twenty years of chronic pain and illness, I have found a life-changing measure of healing—mostly outside of the gauntlet that is modern medicine but still solidly inside the heart of the Catholic Church and God's design for His creation. On one hand, it is an easy story to tell because the foundation of my healing is quite simple. On the other hand, it is full of the daily details of incremental changes, setbacks, and victories. This book will share the keys to that healing with you so that you may likewise be empowered. Making the decision to begin is something that you can do today:

I want you to begin by giving yourself permission to heal. Take that moment right now and embrace the idea that you can and should seek healing!

The decision to begin remains one of the most important moments of my life. I accepted that it was okay for me to invest energy into care of my mind and body so that I could continue to love and serve God and others in my vocation. And because I know that He loves me and He desires that I seek Him in all things.

You can make vital changes even if you have underlying causes which cannot be cured. I want this for you because I see Christ in you. He has given us the Gospel mandate to serve others...so today, I am extending my hand to you. I know that you are sick, grieving, depressed, suffering. It is okay to be weak. He loves you. In His name, will you accept this gift?

The gift is not a silver bullet but an opportunity for transformation. Instead of giving you an effortless miracle (which is quite beyond me anyhow), I'm going to offer you ways to become an advocate for your own health—mind, body, and soul.

THE SIMPLEST PATH

The Sunshine Principle is the simple truth that the greatest potential for healing occurs when we align our behaviors with God's natural, biological, and spiritual laws.

I have witnessed this miracle of design play out in the lives of countless others, and my own story has become a living testimony to God's creative power and love for me. I am the leper and the blind man and the paralytic. If I were to keep silent, the very stones would cry out...and so I write.

When I was 35 years old, I had six children and was suffering through some of the worst pain and sickness of my life. It was the expression of a twenty-year burden, and my body was screeching to a halt.

I had struggled through seven pregnancies and was home-schooling with an aging body, active family, loads of housework, and a husband to love—all the normal obligations of life and the source of my earthly joy. Yet each of these blessings felt like a 100-pound weight on my back reminding me of my failure, and each morning took more courage than I felt I could muster.

For those who have suffered any chronic illness (diagnosed or not),

I don't have to tell you what that burden does to a person. Along with the heaviness of my failures, I trembled at the darkness of my future. I wanted to live but I didn't want to wake up to more pain, and I was certain that I would be in a wheelchair by the time I was forty. I despaired of rising to meet a new day and my very soul felt shackled to pain.

Long I had even considered natural options or writing about natural healing, I reached this crisis point and was truly at the dregs of my courage. I thought I couldn't go on another step, but I took a step anyway and discovered a path to renewed hope and healing. Since then, I have become aware of an epidemic of chronic fatigue, weight loss resistance, pain, and disease among the members of the Body of Christ. Now, I receive numerous email inquiries every day (and I try to answer as many as I can) about my healing testimony. People are suffering and they want to know...

Where do I start? What do I eat? Where do I turn for support? How do I heal in the midst of my suffering and the obligations of my vocation?

I've been there. I *am* there. And taking care of myself is still sometimes a challenging task. I want my experience to help you make the transition much more quickly than I did! I needed this book many times over the years and I pray it is an answer to your need today.

The principles of healing laid out here are straightforward and accessible. They are also fundamentally Catholic in that they honor God's design (as expressed in the natural law and the laws of nature) and are supported by the teachings of the Church. You will find nothing that runs contrary to the faith and, even if you are a non-Catholic Christian, you will be pleased to know that everything is consistent with a Biblical worldview.

My approach avoids beginner burnout by steering clear of specialized details, which can be helpful at later stages but are often too burdensome at the outset. I offer the simplest steps for embarking on the journey toward healing, regardless of your situation. I am not a physician and I don't need to be. **I just want to support individuals and families in their effort to take back control over their own health care in affordable, safe, effective, and natural ways so that**

their "sick care" visits with medical doctors are minimal. I want you to be the CEO of your own health care team ... the healer in your own home.

The chapters that follow are dedicated to the proper under-standing of the role of natural health care in the obligations of our vocation and the exhortations of the Gospel. I explain the Church's position on care of the body in relation to the soul, and the proper way for a Christian to pursue healing while also pursuing holiness. I also offer many simple and practical steps for making these changes while managing common obstacles.

In the "Healing Stories" portion of this book—a precious gem and gift to you from each of the contributors—you will meet men and women (and even a child) who are all on this same journey. Our details differ, our dinner plates and health challenges vary; but I am confident that every reader will find a connection there. These indi-viduals are living proof that faithfulness is consistent with steward-ship of the body and that "health care" is most successful when we are actively involved.

I never realized just how sick I was until I felt well. If God allows me to be sick, I pray that I can peacefully accept this cross and carry it with virtue and grace. However, if my sickness is not God's active will, but is due mainly to my poor dietary choices and lifestyle? Then I wish to set that cross down as quickly as possible to free my arms for service to love.

If you are in the dark night of your health journey and are feeling close to despair, this book is for you. If you are entirely healthy and want to continue with that strength in your future, this book is also for you. And if you are somewhere on the spectrum between those two bookends, trying to navigate a life of self-care while serving others, this book is for you too.

3

WHAT IS NATURAL HEALTH CARE?

Man, though made of body and soul, is a unity. Through his very bodily condition he sums up in himself the elements of the material world. Through him they are thus brought to their highest perfection and can raise their voice in praise freely given to the Creator. For this reason man may not despise his bodily life. Rather he is obliged to regard his body as good and to hold it in honor since God created it and will raise it up on the last day. — *Catechism of the Catholic Church §364*

---

*T*HE PARABLE OF THE TRACTOR

Once upon a time, there were two families who were offered a mission by the governor of their land. He gave them each a good number of acres of fertile fields to sow and to harvest for the benefit of the village and their own families. The crops would be wholesome, nourishing, and delicious; meant to sustain the region's people for service and to bring joy and pleasure to the family table.

Along with the land, the governor presented each family a tractor with which the farmers could do the bulk of the work in the fields. The tractor, explained the landlord, required daily maintenance, but would be an indispensable instrument in accomplishing the mission. Indeed, without this device, the work would be virtually impossible and the crops would die.

The farmers accepted the mission and their tools with enthusiasm and committed themselves to caring for each other, the crops, their tools, and the governor's vision. The work would be demanding and require daily adherence to routine tasks, but they knew that the small acts of faithful obedience would yield abundant fruits.

Seasons came and went, and the families enjoyed plentiful harvests as they toiled energetically toward their goal. They offered prayers of thanksgiving to God every night for the sustenance He so lovingly provided through their generous landlord.

Then disaster struck one of the families. After some thirty years of successful and faithful service, their tractor broke down mid-harvest. The engine refused even to turn over and the family wept as they watched the sun set over their beautiful crops.

The next morning, they brought their tools out to the tractor and applied all of their knowledge and skill to try to get it running. While the machine was not beyond repair, it was unquestionably beyond their ability. The project would require mechanical specialists—parts would need to be ordered and replaced, and there would be no harvest this year. The time delay and costly repairs would make this quite impossible.

The family approached their neighbors, who were busy about their own harvesting, with a plaintive request. *Please, can we borrow your tractor? Ours is broken and we cannot gather our crops.*

The neighboring family looked on them with compassion, but were faced with a dilemma. They were already giving all their time and energy to their own mission. They were charged with the gathering of their own harvest and knew that their tractor (still running strong but also aging) could not handle the work for two families. Besides, their tractor was in use from the break of dawn until darkness covered the land. They generously offered food from their table to support their neighbors but, regrettably, could not help them with the harvest.

Weeks passed and the tractor sat lifeless in the field. The governor visited the family and asked them to account for the great stretch of rotting crops.

"Sir, it is beyond our control. We have no other tractor but the one you provided, and it is broken. We are working with the mechanic but the needed repairs are expensive and complicated."

He said: "I went out to the field to inspect your tractor and found it in poor condition. The filters were clogged and contaminated, the oil dirty and long overdue for a change, the belts and hoses dry, cracked, and failing. You have a corroded fuel line and worn clutch. There is rust everywhere. It's been a long time since daily maintenance or simple repairs were done well. And you have used a cheap fuel for which your machine was not designed."

"But Sir, they protested, we have been so busy about the work that it seemed impossible to tend to all of those things. We have tried to be frugal and delayed costly maintenance. And there were many days when we worked so hard that we had no energy left to attend to duties that could wait for another day. *We worked faithfully to exhaustion for you. We don't know anyone who has worked harder!* And now, the suppliers are slow to ship and the mechanics are overcharging and we cannot afford it. It is an injustice."

And the Governor replied:

"You have only one tractor and now it is broken. I designed it to run with minimal, but essential, daily upkeep. However, you have neglected this gift and now are at the mercy of others to try to fix your errors. Far better for you to have been faithful in the little acts according to my design and preserve the tool so indispensable to your mission. Then, you would only occasionally have need to consult the mechanic for minor repairs. And now you may lose your freedom, livelihood, and ability to complete your mission…"

≈

TENDING YOUR BROKEN TRACTOR

My own "tractor" broke down mid-harvest and I was thrown into a desperate crisis. Many of you are in a similar position—either struggling to bandage your broken body or facing a health crisis at midlife, just when you most need to be active, present, and strong.

Catholics can be inconsistent about health care. Unless we are asking God to grant us a miraculous healing, to bless the hands of the doctors performing surgery, or to give us the grace to suffer well, we tend to separate the practice of health care from the practical application of our faith. We like to talk about "embracing the cross" of our sickness but we don't often talk about the idea that we are the primary caretakers of our bodies and that God designed the created world to support our lives, our health, and our healing.

That is to say, the more closely we align our behaviors and lifestyle choices to God's design for our minds, bodies, and souls, the more fully we can realize healing in all three areas. I do not mean that we should be living in the woods adorned with fig leaves and eating crickets. Rather, that we should be respectfully attentive to immutable biological and theological truths to make the most beneficial choices in our circumstances. Like the "slave to the Truth" of Fr. Sertillanges,[1] the thoughtful, reflective person will intuitively understand the perfect design of God's natural world and will clearly grasp our role in the stewardship of the earth and our bodies.

AM I A "CRUNCHY CATHOLIC"?

Until my 35th year, I was a suburban mom with an aversion to camping, a large collection of toxic cleansers (to accommodate my life of ease), and a lifelong appreciation for junk food. However, I discovered that my food choices and lifestyle were killing me and that I needed to make an immediate and dramatic change. So I added good nutrition and clean living to my growing list of "crunchy" affiliations. My list also included ecological breastfeeding, baby wearing, co-sleeping, bone broth making, and home birthing, among others. But really, I'm still the same suburban mom who enjoys wearing polyester, left my Birkenstocks in the 1990s, and has no serious interest in beekeeping. I even had to teach myself how to eat broccoli at the age of forty.

Nope...not crunchy.

It is tempting to assign ourselves (and others) labels in order to identify and understand. If a label helps you to relate to me, that's fine. But, like all labels, it falls short of conveying the fullness or accuracy of my message.

My name is Melody. I am a child of God made in the Imago Dei, the image of God. My calling is to love and to be loved.

I am a woman who was smacked upside the head with a disease-two-by-four. When that happened, I awakened to the knowledge that God gave me this body as the primary tool of service in my vocation to love and to serve—and I was resolved to fight to restore it to health.

WHAT IS HEALTH CARE?

A standard definition of health might be "the maintenance and improvement of physical and mental health, especially through the provision of medical services."

But, this definition doesn't hold up to practical scrutiny because "medical services" hardly ever address the maintenance portion of a healthy body, only care of a sick one. Ask any physician, and you'll find that the majority of medical school is spent learning to diagnose and treat disease, not to prevent it. Such medical services are typically administered exclusively in a doctor's office or medical facility. Meanwhile, those "maintenance and improvement" services, which actually support our bodies' normal healthy functions are rarely, if ever, covered by "health insurance."

The reality is that the vast majority of our health care should be happening daily in our own homes. Visits to a medical professional should, ideally, be less frequent. The principal responsibility of our health care rests in our own hands—by our prudent practice of Nutrition, Exercise, Rest and Stress Management, Limiting Toxic Exposures, an Active Spiritual Life, and Informed Self-Care. Instead, we often surrender authority over our own health care while we trade our unhealthy lifestyle preferences for a physician's educated guess regarding the source of our ailments. Our reward is a bushel of prescriptions and a mountain of hefty bills.

This book is not about the role that mainstream medical professionals play in the average person's wellness. **There is no question that modern medicine is a blessing when it is needed.** But we have been given great responsibility regarding just when we arrive at that point. This version of health care celebrates our opportunity to become healers in our own homes.

WHAT IS NATURAL HEALTH CARE?

Natural health care is, quite simply, a preference for using those means which are most compatible with and suited to the design of our bodies. If there is an Un-designed Designer, as St. Thomas Aquinas[2] demonstrates, it is only because there is an incontrovertible Design. It is about getting back to biological basics and honoring that original design even while utilizing technological advancements.

As Christians, we believe that God made everything with purpose, and that He intended us to be living tabernacles for Him—indeed, to be His living hands and feet for others by bringing them the Good News of Jesus Christ (Rom. 10:15). Each cell of our bodies has been considered with great love by the Divine Intelligence, Who created the universe. Dismissing natural wellness options is not just short-sighted, but also forgetful of who we are and He Who created us.

God designed the body to eat *real food* (nourishing and compatible with our biology). He designed the body's immune system to keep us healthy. He designed the natural world to perfectly support our needs —all the way down to our mitochondria and DNA. Unfortunately, our fallen culture of self-indulgence and convenience has caused an unprecedented level of sickness in people, animals, and the environment. We are consuming calories which we call "food" but which are non-nutritive and even harmful to the body. We are living in a scenario in which autoimmune disease, allergies, neurological disorders, and cancers are at epidemic proportions and have us desperately scrambling for answers and for healing.

As a culture, we have become detached from knowledge about the beautiful collaboration of our body's systems and have grown to distrust the Creator with our care. Some alarming examples:

- Many women no longer believe that their bodies can safely go into labor or deliver a baby without medical intervention.
- One out of every six Americans is taking a pharmaceutical drug for mental health issues.[3] (and this number is projected to rise.)
- The majority of couples (*including Catholics*) use artificial contraception or even permanent means to destroy healthy fertility.
- Ten percent of deaths (the third highest cause) in the United States are due to medical error which includes fatal pharmaceutical drug reactions.[4]
- Despite superior medical advancements and more money spent on health care, infant mortality in the United States is higher than any other developed nation.[5]
- In spite of a steady decline in the world's maternal mortality rates over a few decades, the U.S. maternal mortality rates have been climbing.[6]

The Church teaches us that every human being is fashioned "in the image of God." Yet, the medical world appears bent on fixing what it sees as inherently flawed about the human design—sometimes before evidence of even a single symptom of dysfunction. And this is in spite of the fact that biological processes, left unhindered but properly supported, will often provide the solution innately. It's not that the original design doesn't work. It is much more likely that we don't understand it, are impatient with the process, or are tempted to tinker in an attempt to make it better.

Has the good Lord really messed up the crowning achievement of his creation so badly that we can look only to the limited science of modern times to save us? Do we really believe that we must correct the mistakes that God made in His creation? And why do we concede such an inexhaustible trust to a system which so often violates Natural Law and even its own ethical standards? Even after allowing for the effects of original sin on the health of our bodies, we add to the burden by regularly ignoring its awesome and correct biological design. This has become the primary reason (after The Fall, of course) that we are suffering with disease.

It may be hard to admit but it's true...

The number one cause of disease in our country is the choices we make—what we do or fail to do in the routine care of our amazing bodies, both individually and generationally. According to the U.S. Center for Disease Control (CDC), the majority of chronic disease in the United States is self-inflicted through poor diet and lifestyle.[7] This is not a secret, and our continued denial will not heal us.

So what will?

4

THE CATHOLIC WAY IS THE NATURAL WAY

I see Jesus in every human being. I say to myself, this is hungry Jesus, I must feed him. This is sick Jesus...I must wash him and tend to him. I serve because I love Jesus. — Saint Teresa of Calcutta

---

*S*ince you have picked up this book, I assume you are at least open to the idea that natural healing can be consistent with a life of faith...and you're absolutely right! There is nothing good in our health care industry which is not ultimately acquired from the gifts of creation and, consequently, from God. The Catholic way of natural healing does not exclude authentic advancements of science, but seeks a path of harmony with science which most closely honors the dignity and biology of the body.

We may think of our local Catholic parish as a sort of spiritual hospital where we seek solace and healing primarily for the immortal soul. However, we discover that we are compelled to enter with our bodies still attached to our souls. That is part of the mystery and beauty of our humanity. There is not a dichotomy, but a magnificent and preordained harmony between the spiritual and the physical. The body is animated by the soul, and the soul will (eventually) be joined to the body forever. It is the only way because it is the way we are made. It is the way Christ chose for Himself and for us. We do not believe, as do some Eastern religions, that the body is just a hindrance to the spiritual. Rather, we know that the body is precious—because it houses the reflection of the majesty and love of God—and is the means by which we become holy.

There is no contradiction between the desire to be well and the desire to serve the Lord. As believers, we are frequently willing to "offer it up" when we suffer. Why is it so difficult, then, to "offer up" the discipline it takes to stay healthy? We take up the crosses intended for our sanctification and then, because we have free will and an insatiable appetite for goodies (St. Thomas called them 'apparent goods'), we decide to pick up a few additional crosses that don't (and shouldn't) belong to us. Oddly enough, we sometimes even design and build our own crosses, fit them carefully to our shoulders, and then struggle under the grievous weight. *I'm sorry, Lord. I want to do more for you but...my tractor is broken.*

GRACE AND NATURE

The tradition of the Church acknowledges two kinds of healing power: grace and nature. We read from the Congregation for the Doctrine of the Faith:

Obviously, recourse to prayer does not exclude, but rather encourages the use of effective natural means for preserving and restoring health, as well as leading the Church's sons and daughters to care for the sick, to assist them in body and spirit, and to seek cure disease. [1]

As the hands and feet of Christ, we serve others and seek to remain fit for that life of service. As the brothers and sisters of Christ, we must also allow others to care for us—remembering that we are the "the least of these" whom God loves (Matt 25:40). It is His will that we be treated with dignity and love, body and soul. God's gifts of healing are for you and me, and there should be no shame or guilt in seeking what God provides, only gratitude and faithfulness. The CDF continues:

The Fathers of the Church considered it normal that believers would ask God not only for the health of their soul, but also for that of their body. With regard to the goods of life, health, and physical integrity, St. Augustine writes: 'We need to pray that these are retained, when we have them, and that they are increased, when we do not have them.

THE OBLIGATION TO PURSUE NATURAL SOLUTIONS

Rational acceptance of the order of nature...is at the same time recognition of the right of the Creator. — Karol Wojtyla, *Love and Responsibility*

Our aspiration to find more, discover more, cure more, and create more may provide additional insights into God's design, but they do not elevate us to the status of co-designer. Nor should they fill us with the silly notion that we can do better. So beguiled at first by our own invention, we are often later astonished to find that the original design was best after all. Sometimes our tinkering even damages more than it cures. Instead of cooperating, we have co-opted. We spend an inordinate amount of money and time figuring out how to forestall death and avoid discomfort. The greater part of our resources should be given to simply honoring God's design.

We will still suffer the wages of sin, we will experience pain, and we will die. But, along the way, we can remain fit for service in the kingdom and honor God by treating His creation (our own bodies and souls) with the same level of care, tenderness, and reverence as He would. Given man's failures in this regard, it is no wonder that the great moral issues of our time are inseparable from the struggle of orienting our behavior to the laws of our biological design: Marriage & Sexuality, Conception & Contraception, Childbirth & Abortion, Euthanasia & Assisted Suicide.

Human health depends upon alignment with God's design and the principle of subsidiarity (CCC 1883-1885). In every case, a departure from natural and biological law results in a distortion of the goodness intended for humanity—temporally and sometimes eternally. Classically, this distortion of the good is called evil.

Because we are sinners, it is not difficult for us to lose touch with God's truth, which is revealed through nature and our God-breathed design. It takes a conscious effort (and sometimes an all-out battle) to retain or re-educate ourselves about who we are and the connection between God's design and salvation.

NATURAL AND BIOLOGICAL LAW

The natural law, present in the heart of each man and established by reason, is universal in its precepts and its authority extends to all men. It expresses the dignity of the person and determines the basis for his fundamental rights and duties. — Catechism of the Catholic Church §1965

Broadly, natural law refers to inherently known principles that reflect the Divine Law and which govern the behavior of mankind with respect to God's creation. The natural law is an expression of the unchanging truth of God's plan for creation written on our minds and hearts and knowable by all people through the light of natural reason. Part of natural law governs human biology in the sense that how we treat ourselves—what kinds of diet, rest, exercise and the like we choose—has both physical and spiritual (or moral) consequences.

Clearly, the Church's tradition does not sanction many of the current cultural fads. Instead, it addresses the truth that God's creation provides us with goodness and healing. In Love and Responsibility, Karol Wojtyla (the future Pope St. John Paul II) wrote: "Man's actions must be in harmony with the laws of nature." Perhaps this explains why so many families have an idyllic vision of a home with a little bit of land, a garden, and some chickens. Our very souls seem to yearn for a slower pace and closer proximity to the natural world.

St. Thomas Aquinas tells us that nature must, in a sense, become our teacher since it reveals the creativity, intellect, and will of Almighty God:

And so in the things that it makes, the human intellect, which derives the light of intelligence from the divine intellect, must be informed by the examination of the things that come about through nature so that it may operate in the same way. — St. Thomas Aquinas, *Commentary on Aristotle's Politics, prologue*

We take seriously the counsel of The Angelic Doctor, but not always. On one hand, practicing Catholics accept the sometimes-challenging teaching of the Church that we must follow the biological laws governing human sexuality. On the other, by our actions we reject the idea that those same biological laws can impact other ordinary functions of our lives—such as eating, drinking, farming, exercising, medicating, and producing material goods. However, the cause-and-effect principles inherent in God's design—as evident in the processes of human sexuality, childbirth, care of the newborn and the elderly—also apply to the general care of the body which is made in the *Imago Dei*.

We read in *Evangelium Vitae* ("The Gospel of Life"), that every human being is "an icon of Jesus Christ," and "a sign of the living God," and "the image of God's glory" (n 84). In light of that awesome mystery, we should reflect carefully on the way that we treat our bodies. Unfortunately, it is often only in the later stages of disease and distress that we understand how our choices have negatively impacted our ability to serve.

Is this a moral issue? Absolutely! We care for the unborn, the newly born, the young, and the elderly. Why do we so sorely neglect the ages in between? Are we not also worthy of a similar dignity and safekeeping? Are we not charged with the care of those around us? If our lifestyle choices are rendering us less able to serve others, how can it be anything but a moral issue?

I cannot offer the perfect path to wellness for your body, nor do I claim to know the degree to which you should pursue that goal. Instead, I want to encourage, educate, and empower you to advocate for and discern the role you ought to play in your own healing.

APPLYING THE PRINCIPLE OF SUBSIDIARITY

You wish to reform the world? Reform yourself, otherwise your efforts will be in vain. — St. Ignatius of Loyola

---

The principle of subsidiarity is among the most important concepts with respect to health and wellness since it honors the basic principles of freedom. Generally, it holds that practical decision-making should always happen at the lowest possible level at which it can be done effectively. Subsidiarity is frequently used with respect to political systems, wherein it calls for the greatest possible participation at the level closest to home. This provides for a higher degree of accountability and the protection of human dignity and the common good.

How does this relate to health care? As our hospital systems grow, health insurance becomes more complex, and available medical care becomes largely dictated by for-profit pharmaceutical and insurance companies. The food industry also gains growing control over our nutrition options as some large corporate interests have been granted immunity from legal responsibility, even from manifestly negligent actions. This subjugation of fundamental human need to political interests puts us at frightening risk of losing active participation in and any control over some of the most essential aspects of our lives.

The implementation of basic principles of subsidiarity in health care can change our culture, our world, and the Church. In practical terms, this is a return to the cardinal rules of health care (guided, unsurprisingly, by the Cardinal Virtues) and keeping as many people as possible under the care of the family or those closest to the family.

The most obvious example is nutrition (or lack thereof), which is the root cause (or cure) for a multitude of modern ailments. If I have burdened myself with preventable diabetes through hundreds of poor choices over time, I have surrendered much of my health care freedom. If I do not choose wisely in favor of health, I will become dependent on a system of pharmaceutical and surgical care. Ultimately, I make the choice whether or not to surrender these freedoms and preferences in the way I make daily health decisions. For instance, where I could previously have decided, "I choose not to eat a second helping of ice cream," I now must say "I cannot eat any ice cream at all," or, "I can only have ice cream along with this medication that will prevent a diabetic emergency."

The great news is that, even in sickness, we can often regain some of that freedom by making fundamental changes. This can be difficult to believe when physicians decree certain illnesses "incurable," or don't offer alternatives to life-long dependence on pharmaceuticals. Even more unbelievable is the fact that so many physicians do not offer these alternatives.

There are five primary reasons why traditional doctors will not recommend or refer for alternatives:

- First, many physicians have not been educated in nutrition beyond a cursory treatment. They are not generally taught about nutrition as a viable path for managing disease and symptoms.[2]
- Second, many are limited by financial pressures or employers' insistence to follow a pharmaceutical model.
- Third, the life experience of the typical physician tells them that the patient—the 21st century American who is accustomed to luxury and averse to change—will likely choose to take medication rather than adjust a lifestyle, so they may consider the effort wasted.
- Fourth, they are afraid of getting sued or running into legal trouble for recommending alternatives to medications.
- Fifth, they simply don't have time to teach their patients the fundamental building blocks of good health, which do not require a medical degree to learn and implement.

The foregoing does not imply that the average physician is a bad person or an incompetent professional, but it does highlight the need to be conscious of our responsibility for our own care and the limitations of the system. **Culpability for unhealthy habits and poor nutrition does not ultimately fall at the feet of the physician.**

For fifteen years, I was tossed from one medical specialist to another, and not one of them suggested dietary changes. The sad truth is that I had at my disposal the tools to change my life that entire time. My mistake was relying on doctors to fix what was really my responsibility. In my defense, I was a product of the culture and simply "didn't know what I didn't know." I was also unaware that my body was struggling with a tremendous burden from undiagnosed disease.

My own renewal has been realized, not through the medical system (under which I got progressively sicker), but through the encouragement of friends, and even through some of the much-maligned but popular internet personalities. These folks gave me some free tools that no physician seemed capable of providing for many thousands of dollars.

The only real hope for a large-scale culture of healing is for individuals to start taking a passionate interest in their own well-being—choosing to be alert, active, and free instead of living in bondage to unhealthy relationships with food and unnecessary medication—and waging a never-ending battle with disease.

I would be remiss if I didn't acknowledge all of the amazing, hard-working, virtuous physicians and medical professionals who truly have a heart for helping their patients heal—the ones whose compassion for their suffering patients allows them to resist the temptation to play God. I want to acknowledge and bless those good men and women who fight the inclination to become jaded and, instead, trust people to make good decisions. I want to encourage those professionals who have the humility to accept that there may be another way, even if they don't know what it is. All of these wonderful people in health care are certainly doing the Lord's work.

I also want to express my gratitude to the doctors who are blazing the trail for functional and integrative medicine around the world. As pioneers, they are often misunderstood, but their patients (including me) know that they are meeting a need that is deep and wide. They are taking a risk to help build a healthier and happier life for each soul they touch.

IS THAT YOUR CROSS?

Men are generally the carpenters of their own crosses.
— St. Philip Neri

Soon after I started sharing my health challenges and healing efforts online, the emails began to pour in. In fact, the requests for help were so numerous that I retreated a bit because I could not keep up with the flood of messages. I did not want people to feel that I was ignoring or abandoning them in their need. Most of them were variations on a story:

I am overwhelmed by the burden of my own failure. I am exhausted. I am sick. My weight has skyrocketed. My stomach hurts, my body is on fire with pain, and my doctor can't help me. My life is one-step-forward-two-steps-back and my relationships are floundering. I wake up every morning feeling just as hopeless as I felt the night before.

The palpable grief and hopelessness in these stories affects me deeply, and this is why I am sticking my little neck out in an expert-saturated world. If you have reached out to me at some point and I have failed you, please know I regret my inadequacy and that I am praying for you. This book is the email I wanted to send you and the phone conversation I wanted to have with you.

I reject the notion that you are a horrible failure at life. I think you probably have critical human needs that are not being met. In our relative wealth, we tend to look with pity and compassion on those in physically impoverished nations, and have at least some awareness of our own privilege. What we fail to truly grasp is that, **along with a depth of spiritual impoverishment in Western nations, we are also experiencing a crisis of physical impoverishment.** Perhaps this is because we are so aware of the abundant blessings in our lives and our almost utter lack of want for any material need, especially as compared with our brothers and sisters who live in destitution.

Ironically, even the well-fed among us end up with variations of the same diseases that afflict the malnourished and indigent: respiratory complications, nutrient deficiencies, infection and parasitic disease, and poor maternal and neonatal outcomes. Add the illnesses more common to developed countries, which include cancers, diabetes, neuropsychiatric disorders, cardiovascular disease, autoimmune dysfunction, and digestive disease. The list begins to take on staggering proportions.

We are no longer a collection of healthy communities supporting the sick. We now seem rather like chronically sick communities living on pharmaceuticals and addictions (social media, noise, distractions, drugs, coffee, alcohol, etc.) in order to "get by."

As Catholics, we are called to embrace a pro-life worldview of natural, biologically-consistent health care. The alternative is falling complacently into the enemy's trap of persistent physical, mental, and emotional isolation.

Is that the cross God is asking you to carry? Or is He waiting for you to set down that artificial tree in order that you may take up the beautiful cross of your greater life work? I don't expect to ever be fully free from suffering in this life, but I have discovered that a simple change in lifestyle sets me free from some of those self-inflicted crosses so that I have the strength to carry the ones truly belonging to my state in life.

If your cross is of your own making, set it down. The whole point of this exercise is to become renewed for God's service—free to serve. Not just for you, but to teach future generations how to build a culture which honors personal dignity for the greater glory of God.

GENERATIONAL HEALING

After the New York legislature passed a bill legalizing abortion up to birth, a social media commentator observed that, "It seems the more we advance medically, the more we return to the barbarisms abandoned a millennia ago." This "slouching towards Gomorrah"[3] is an unambiguous danger as we allow incremental changes to slowly strip us of our connection to God. This is often the path of evil—it seeks to separate us from the love of God by separating us from His truth. It starts small until we become acclimated to a change and then it presses forward more boldly over time. We often recognize this in the most grievous offenses like abortion, but fail to see it in the seemingly trivial daily habits, which slowly destroy our bodies, our mental acuity, and our relationships.

Years ago, I made a cake from a popular 1950s cookbook I thrifted from a neighborhood garage sale. The recipe was touted as "best ever!" Upon sampling it, we were more than a little surprised to find that the dense texture and bland taste were not at all pleasant. We had been so conditioned to the taste of fluffy boxed cake mixes that, when we cooked with whole ingredients, we didn't like it. Our appetites have been systematically directed by an industry that profits by consistent results and predictable taste. Not every reader may see that as a bad thing, but we can't deny the impact of industrialized preferences that have been guided and shaped by commercial agendas.

Somewhere in the last few generations, we have collectively come to accept that pre-packaged, chemically enhanced boxed meals are the normal delivery method for meals. We applaud our ingenuity and affluence in creating such convenient tasty choices. We allow marketing to dictate our food selections and our preferences for sweets to dictate the health of our bodies. We have accepted that preparing nutritional food every day is "too difficult" and we don't even realize that the chain of generational memory—the passing on of knowledge from one generation to the next—has been broken.

In *The Way of Beauty*, author David Clayton writes :

If the man-made environment participates in that pattern of divine wisdom too, then we have an environment that will be a constant influence that educates those who live there whether they are aware of it or not.[4]

Clayton was referring here to architecture and the importance of creating a beautiful environment, reflecting the beauty of the cosmos as a physical manifestation of divine wisdom. I believe we can extrapolate and identify similar principles in the other areas of our lives. For instance, recognizing such things as beautiful movement and beautiful food, in that they reflect divine wisdom and work to our greatest good. We are now starting to see how our interference in that wisdom is harming us: physically, environmentally, socially, and spiritually. Advancements in medicine, food production, and communication have brought new sets of problems that, ironically, seem to be making us sicker and more isolated than ever. In seeking to improve upon previous generations, much wisdom has been lost. Our ability to course-correct is hampered as generations are beguiled by ubiquitous technology. Fewer grandmothers are teaching the art of food preparation because they grew up on boxed meals. Fewer grandfathers are mentoring about home maintenance because too much of their youth was spent in front of the TV.

We live in a world that is alive with the awesome expression of God's magnanimous creativity, and yet we have fed ourselves into a stupor of gluttonous standardization. Part of my mission and hope is to publicly acknowledge these broken connections and call for restoration and a proper use of our freedom. There is risk in freedom. There is also the possibility for discovering the holy and wild gift of creation, made for our benefit.

Leila Marie Lawler, popular Catholic writer at "Like Mother, Like Daughter," speaks regularly about the importance of healing the "collective memory" in our families. She shared with me:

The collective memory is the wisdom that is passed from one generation to the next without necessarily being written down. It's the culture—the beautiful WAY of living the truth that arises from the "cult"—the worship of the people. It concerns spiritual things but also simple, mundane ways of living and doing. Not everything can be learned from a book! Some things must be learned from experience and observation and art. Women are the guardians of this type of memory, in large part —hence the term "old wives' tale"—now used in derision, but not lightly to be dismissed!

The collective memory is the wisdom about life that we don't want to lose. Since our own culture is about rejecting all that is in the past and making all things new and from nothing, this memory is lost or in danger of being lost. Even knowing that these things should be kept is a bit of wisdom to hold on to!

In my own family, I hope to restore a little of what has been lost. This book is part of the legacy of health and hope that I want to weave into the collective memory of my family and community—to strengthen the Body of Christ in service, equipped for the crosses that are inevitably in store. I know, unfortunately, that my bad choices have contributed to generational wounds—physically, spiritually, and emotionally. These pages are part of the legacy of generational healing which I feel compelled to pass on to those entrusted to my care.

DO YOU WANT TO BE HEALED?

When Jesus saw him and knew that he had been lying there a long time, he said to him, 'do you want to be healed? — John 5:6

Shortly after my lupus diagnosis, I was at a large pro-life event sharing my story of healing with people who stopped by my table. I spoke in general terms, but when the larger crowd drifted away, one woman remained. She asked me about myself and I gave her a few more details.

"I have lupus..."

Her eyes narrowed and she adopted what I can only call a fighting stance. She spoke deliberately and with strength:

You don't have lupus! And lupus don't have you! What you have is a body that thinks it needs to attack itself in order to survive and that involves a WHOLE lot of mess. But don't you name it! I don't want to hear that from your mouth again. Don't you give something that don't exist power over you. You've got symptoms. And you told me yourself that you intend to heal. So put that diagnosis down! I know it's easier to use a word to explain what's happening to you. But in your own head, you've got to know that you are free to heal.

Then she left.

I've been unpacking that short speech ever since, and her words have permanently altered my outlook on illness. I still use the word "lupus" because it is convenient and quickly communicates some specifics to others. Conversations get ridiculously long if I explain things her way! But adjusting my inner dialogue has changed the way I approach autoimmune disease and I am grateful that she challenged me.

She was right. I have a collection of symptoms that are the result of a confused immune system, and everything in my healing toolbox right now is focused on eliminating the cause of the problem and healing the damage. It is when I start to focus too much on "lupus" that I begin to despair. A diagnosis can be beneficial, but it can also be a chimera. Focusing too intently on the eradication of the diagnosis, rather than the healing of my body, can easily distract me from the most biologically beneficial healing actions.

According to most medical authorities, lupus is an incurable disease, which requires harmful and complicated pharmaceuticals in order to manage. It is similar to cancer, in that harm must often be done to the body in order to help heal the body. If my disease is only about the lupus diagnosis, then that is my fate, to hopefully delay death and disability from disease (or from medication).

But if I recognize that there is an underlying reason that my antibodies continuously assault my own body, then I have a chance of not only improving my symptoms, but also of eradicating the diagnosis entirely.

I have been part of several online support forums filled with people who believe that they can never be well. That may be true and it may not be, but we must hear and answer the question the Lord himself has asked a dying man (John 5:6) and answer this question boldly and faithfully:

Do you want to be well?

Yes! Most emphatically, yes. For the sake of my family and if it is the will of God, please Jesus, give me the desire and the means to be well!

5

READY TO HEAL? START HERE

I have heard your prayer, I have seen your tears; behold, I will heal you...
— 2 Kings 20:5

I often hear from readers who are looking for healing and a new beginning and who aren't sure where to start. Our stories, while varied and unique, are generally defined by a few shared, basic difficulties: we are sick, we are tired, we are overwhelmed, and we need help.

First, I want to say THANK YOU to all who heroically embrace your call to serve, even while laboring under the burden of your private (and often invisible) suffering. I'm not going to make light of the suffering you bear. I'm not going to lie and say that this is going to be a breeze. However, there is a way. There are specific steps which will make the journey easier and more joyful. When in doubt (and when exhausted), revisit these key steps, make a small movement, and claim the victory.

1. STAY ROOTED IN THE HEART OF CHRIST.

Just as He was with the Apostles on the Sea of Galilee, Jesus is here with us in the midst of the storm. We may be afraid, but remember that He is in control. When the time is right, He will say, "Peace, Be Still," and the winds will die down and the water will calm. The struggle is here to stay, at least for a time, and we will have to rely on His Presence in sacrament and prayer for hope and sustenance. Your body is His creation and He loves you. Stay close to Him always and be encouraged. I recommend that you start this journey (and every day) with prayer that includes the following elements, and with an emphasis on *constant* expressions and acts of gratitude:

- Repentance
- Forgiveness of others and self
- Petition for healing and mercy
- Acceptance of the will of God
- Thanksgiving
- Adoration

2. CLEAR YOUR CALENDAR.

You cannot heal if your schedule excludes healing activities. If you think that you cannot make time for these things now, imagine the difficulty you will face when you will be forced to make time in the midst of a health crisis. Stop guiltily hoarding moments of solace and begin building healthy space into the very rhythm of your family life. If that means hiding out in your bedroom periodically, accept it, and don't allow the blessing of a healing intermission to be sabotaged by useless guilt. Maintaining a holy pace of life (one which promotes health of mind, body, and soul) is not shameful but should be encouraged and protected.

3. DEFINE YOUR DREAM

A few years ago, I attended an Arise retreat with fifty other women. I will never forget the day that the retreat master tackled the pain of womanhood head-on. He spoke to our sense of failure, our self- loathing, our heartbreaks, and then he asked us:

Ladies, where is your joy? Where are your dreams? You were created to be the guardians of joy...arise!

Audible gasps erupted in the room from the "guardians of joy," so heavily burdened by mountains of failure and grief. He had shot an arrow straight into the epicenter of our pain and simultaneously opened a door that many of us had considered permanently closed. In an attempt to protect ourselves from more pain, we had accepted a life of limitation and closed ourselves off to healing and joy. Many of us were carrying a burden of sorrow which was interfering with our ability to love and serve. It is one thing to suffer well—we *will* suffer and we ought to do it well! It is another thing to live with a spirit of hopelessness and grief. Sometimes we just need to be reminded that we are allowed—*called*—to dream and to reach for something beautiful; and that holiness is not an oppressor but a fire lighted by the Divine.

A few years ago, my 'unattainable dream' was simply to sleep, move, and eat without agony. Repeated failure was too painful and I almost gave up hope. My vision of heaven was as a giant exit button rather than a joyful union. My dreams were little more than a desperate cry for release. Slowly, God helped me to relax my clenched fists and open my eyes. I had been in a defensive posture for so long that dreaming again was as terrifying as standing on the precipice of an ocean cliff. My terror eventually gave way to relief and the door to healing was opened.

The process has not been quick or easy, but one of the most significant healing changes I have experienced over the last several years has been a release from the grip of hopelessness and fear. With that release, I have also been able to embrace a return of dreams, a restoration of youthfulness of spirit even in the presence of suffering, and a renewed longing for Christ. My physical healing was a catalyst for every other kind of healing. Some may see that as a sign of my spiritual immaturity, and I cannot disagree. But I was not strong enough to lift (or lower) myself to a better place. I was not capable of saving myself. God saw my distress and provided the means for me to heal in the ways that were necessary for my soul. I don't question His ways...I just give thanks.

What is your dream? It's okay if it is small. Write it down. Say it out loud. Give it to God and let Him lead you.

4. START LEARNING

I intend for this book to meet readers at the first checkpoint of understanding how to heal in the midst of the storm. Take it one step at a time. Start learning about yourself and your goals, about the wisdom that the Church has to offer, and about what it's going to take for you to begin. And then keep going. Become the CEO of your health care.

5. CHOOSE ONE THING AT A TIME AND DO IT.

A wise person once said: "There's more reality in slicing carrots than in discoursing about carrots." That neatly sums up our 'little way" to healing! Take one step forward even when it's hard and count it a victory. In the book *The Slight Edge*, Jeff Olson bluntly writes:

It's easy to eat well. But it's also easy not to, and to go on eating the food that will eventually kill us, because it won't kill us today. It's not the one junk food meal; it's the thousands, over time....And not eating it won't transform your health and save your life, at least not today. Compounded over time, it can and it will.

He makes a simple but powerful point about why so many in our fast-food, click-bait culture don't reach their goals—because they aren't willing to do the one mundane, easy thing in the moment, without experiencing immediate results. In the wise words of St. Therese of Lisieux: "Do small things with great love and do them well." She did not promise an immediate reward, nor should we expect one.

One day at a time, one choice at a time. Step by step. Progress is rarely quick, effortless, or linear. But then one day, you have turned a corner (physically, mentally, or spiritually) and you find yourself standing in the middle of the produce department bawling like a baby and thanking God, because you remember a time when you were too sick to go on short shopping trips with your husband. Yes, that happened to me. That day in the grocery store was when it all made sense; the day I knew that every little positive choice had been worth it. Slowly, steadily, faithfully. That's how lives are transformed.

6. FOCUS ON THE IMMUNE SYSTEM

Your immune system is the bedrock of your physical health, and everything in this book is written to help you get it back in working order. Everything you eat, breathe, do, think, or speak has a direct impact on your immune health. If you yell frequently in anger, you are increasing your stress hormones and depressing your immune system. When you eat, you are directly impacting inflammation levels in your body and harming or improving your gut health, which is the location of the bulk of your body's immune arsenal.

How you sleep, what medications you take, how often you are hugged, how often you pray...every detail in your life impacts your immune health and cooperates with (or opposes) God's design for your body. When it comes to caring for yourself, simply do the next best thing for the foundation of your body's health. It may be as uncomplicated as stepping outside for a walk in the fresh air.

7. BE PATIENT

Healing is rarely a well-paved, direct highway. It is more like a winding journey of successes and setbacks. That's okay. If you are sick, it probably took a long time for your body to get to this point, and it will also likely take time to heal. Hang in there and cling to the goodness of God's design for His sake. Rest if you need to, but don't quit.

God's delays are mysterious; [...] God may abstain for the moment from healing, not because Love does not love, but because Love never stops loving, and a greater good is to come from the woe. Heaven's clock is different from ours. —Venerable Fulton Sheen

---

8. STUBBORNLY NURTURE HOPE

Let it be said of you that you were stubbornly attached to fighting for goodness until God called you home. Refuse to quit fighting, even if it means the sacrifice that you offer is lying in bed sick for a month with no progress on your to-do list. Recommit every day to finding the joy, the victory, and the hope.

You can win some battles even if all odds are against you—even if disease seems to be drawing the very life from you. And when you have reached the end of your physical stamina, that spark will remain as you allow your soul to complete the victory in Christ Jesus.

You cannot lose. He has already won the victory for you. It is a radical notion. It is your destiny as a Christian.

With that victory anthem in mind, I have one more secret to success in your healing journey. It is, in my opinion, the most important.

9. GRATITUDE: THE NON-NEGOTIABLE KEY TO SUCCESS

Every once in a while, I find myself on the receiving end of a look that expresses both bewilderment and admiration. "I don't know how you do it," I'll hear. "I couldn't do what you do." I don't deserve the implied compliment and I certainly don't want to lead anyone to believe that I am doing something astonishing or incredible. So I answer truthfully:

I don't have great willpower. If I eat one chip, I end up eating them all. What I do have is gratitude. Everything changed when I stopped looking at my lifestyle as a series of losses and instead saw each choice as a gift of healing from God.

The moment I start to throw a pity-party about the things I don't get to have is the moment I lose. Nurturing regret creates a false sense of entitlement to the comforts of life. It promotes a selfish mindset and makes gratitude impossible. It also places the missing object of desire in the front of the mind, making it almost impossible to be at peace emotionally until we possess it.

Gratitude, on the other hand, releases us from bondage to our self-ishness. We might be tempted to feel victimized by our losses—subjected to a perceived injustice. But there is no injustice in skipping, or even being denied, a donut. When I am hanging out at a 'Donut Sunday' after Mass, I decide not to become emotionally involved in the loss and I retreat to the refuge and essential habit of thanking God.

"Thank you, Lord, for this parish family. Thank you for the strength to be present here this Sunday. Thank you for the scent of the donuts...they smell delicious. Thank you for showing me a path to healing. Thank you for the opportunity to grow stronger in so many ways. Thank you for vegetables!"

I pray that prayer for as long as it takes. Even if it is sometimes forced or comical, that prayer becomes a habit of actively cultivating gratitude and peace. Like a muscle that gets stronger each time it is used, virtue grows more powerful and stable each time it is exercised.

In order to succeed, you must adopt a spirit of gratitude! It is the indispensable aspect of long-term healing. It won't always (or even usually) flow from warm fuzzy emotion, and you will have to consciously look at Christ and acknowledge the truth. Each time you speak the truth through Him it will strengthen your resolve. Pursue habits of goodness (virtue) and reject habits of self-destruction (vice).

Choose to change that one habit now and you will change everything. How would your life transform if you took delight in God's gifts for you, even when they look more like broccoli than like donuts? There are many people who would rather surrender their health and lives (by a thousand small choices) rather than forgo a handful of luxuries.

God doesn't love you more because He gives you access to cookies, and He doesn't love others less because they live in poverty. His ways are mysterious but His love is consistent, passionate, and unmerited. It is a grave tragedy when we refuse those gifts by building a wall of ingratitude around our hearts and minds.

I was only able to change my behavior when I decided that I would not live another day in my repository of self-pity. I would no longer whine about what I couldn't have. He allowed me to feel enough pain to be willing to break out of old habits and forge new ones.

"ENOUGH!" I cried. "It is enough. I am ready to grow. There are now things that I want more than I want donuts. Thank you. Thank you. Thank you."

Are you ready? Say it out loud: "Thank you, Jesus." Now...let's keep going.

6

HEALING THE BODY

Do you not know that your body is a temple of the Holy Spirit within you, which you have from God? You are not your own; you were bought with a price. So glorify God in your body. — 1 Corinthians 6:19-20

---

*I*t often seems that the story of my personal journey is repeated back to me many times through the words of others: "I got away with poor nutrition, sedentary lifestyle, and a toxic physical environment for years—decades even—but now my body is broken and I can't function."

I want you to know that I thoroughly understand, and I wish to share an important lesson that I have learned: *Wine and Starbucks will only take you so far. The popular understanding of self-care often only delays the inevitable, and is nothing more than a long-term recipe for pain and illness.*

Our splurges and comforts may temporarily numb the pain or mimic vitality, but they do not actually heal, nourish, or strengthen.

Fortunately, for most of us, there is a way to rise to a place that isn't perpetual survival mode. Healing does not exclude suffering, and suffering doesn't exclude healing. A healthy pursuit of virtue will include a Christ-centered embrace of both.

I'm prioritizing my health so that I can serve my family for the rest of my life and continue to raise children for the next twenty years and beyond. When I am troubled by the notion that this prioritization is a selfish and imbalanced goal, I am quickly reminded that I have no other viable choice. Nor do I wish to carry burdens that aren't of God, that I have placed upon my own shoulders through poor or sloppy choices, or that a little discipline will eliminate.

For me, this renewal will not be found in a margarita or ice cream splurge, but in radical lifestyle change. I have already begun, but the race is far from finished. It is a beautiful gift to me from God...and also my gift back to Him.

The struggle has taught me many things about my body, but primarily the following: that nourishing food is a key component to a happy, healthy life; that a wholesome environment is integral to a healthy mind and body; and that a lifestyle absent good nutrition, regular movement, and healthy environment frequently leads to illness and depression.

Because of my experiences of suffering, I became more aware of the suffering of others around me and was surprised by how many people were going through similar things. But I was even more surprised to see that it wasn't just moms with many children who were fatigued and sick—it was also young and single men and women, fathers with blue- and white-collar jobs, children, grandparents, the poor and the wealthy, college students, physicians, farmers, teachers, and even fitness professionals.

We push ourselves to do what needs doing. We brace ourselves for the pain. We learn to live with less sleep. We gain some weight. We lose some strength. We eat cold chicken nuggets that our kids leave on their plates and drain another cup of coffee to keep up the pace.

We learn about our hidden strengths and that our limits expand when we push against them. We learn that it feels good to stretch in service of Truth and Beauty and that our deepest joy is found in that service! We are grateful, joyful, trusting, and prayerful. We learn to push through, in "survival mode," to get to the other side.

But we also know that there are physical laws which govern our bodies, and that there are limits which cannot be breached without harm. It may take a while, but eventually we all learn the hard truth about our earthly existence...

Our bodies have limits. And some of us are breaking.

You have been called to preach the Gospel with your life and that makes care of your body an obligation. But this is not a gloomy journey, or a journey of loss. It is a journey of JOY and of stretching to uncover a little more of the beauty God has chosen for your life! I am a living testimony that our small choices can become great miracles. And I'm actively walking, sometimes crawling, and even (occasionally) running the path with you.

One of the foundational truths that is crucial to embracing a healing lifestyle is that our body is created in love, for love, and by love. As St. Thomas Aquinas wrote: "Grace does not destroy nature, but perfects it." **The body itself is not an obstacle to happiness, but the chosen vehicle for God's plan of eternal joy.**

YOUR BODY IS NOT THE ENEMY

The human person, created in the image of God, is a being at once corporeal and spiritual, Man, whole and entire, is therefore willed by God. — Catechism of the Catholic Church §362

When I was a young girl, I despised my body and often avoided looking in a mirror because the image was a reminder that I was unlovable. I thought I was ugly in every way. I was encouraged in that false belief by every movie and magazine cover which offered only images of people in a state of physical perfection. I also often felt stupid around my peers and frequently counted my faults and awkward missteps well into the night.

Consequently, I was consoled by and attracted to the New Age idea that our bodies are essentially an obstacle to happiness. I fell into the Manichean error that the spiritual world was light and good and the physical world was dark and evil. I hated my physicality and couldn't wait to be 'free' of it forever. I would fly away in my mind from the feeling of being tied down to the earth by this dead fleshy weight.

Satan takes particular demonic delight in accusing young ladies of these lies.

You are dumb. Ugly. Chubby. Awkward. Worthless.

Those meditations led me to an even deeper involvement in non-Christian spirituality, in which I sought to unite myself more closely to the 'universe' and farther away from earth. As a result, I had physical and emotional experiences of apparent tranquility surrounded by what I thought were other seeking souls (but which I now know were demonic). Those spiritual excursions became like a drug to me as I spent more time and effort trying to achieve them. However, they didn't make me more at peace with life, but less so. I became increasingly comfortable with the notion of suicide because I saw it as a stepping out into a peaceful nothingness. I didn't really want to die. I simply wanted to be free of my body.

The roots of those feelings are complex. The result of those feelings was a desire to self-harm, starve, and disappear. The ephemeral serenity I had experienced during new age meditations was quickly replaced by shrill indictments and mental torments that I could not turn off. Unfortunately, I think my experience is somewhat common. Although not everyone experiences demonic attacks so directly, the enemies of God clearly seek to destroy goodness and true peace, and to cause a person to have an unholy hatred of their very flesh—which has been fashioned in the holy Image of God and by His loving hands.

The worldly solutions to such feelings of ugliness and pain are to escape from, punish, or perfect the body. This easily leads to a culture of self-harm or, on the opposite end of the spectrum, a cult of the body which seeks perfection through flawless physical appearance or incomparable athletic achievement. What is lacking in all of these errors, and what ultimately saved my life, was an understanding of the gift of my body through God's eyes and the life-giving teachings of the Catholic faith.

In the Catechism, we read:

---

§2289 *Morality requires respect for the life of the body, it does not make it an absolute value. It rejects a neo-pagan notion that tends to promote the cult of the body, to sacrifice everything for its sake, to idolize physical perfection and success at sports. By its selective preference of the strong over the weak, such a conception can lead to the perversion of human relationships.*

Until adulthood, I floundered between this cult of the body and the opposing view that the body itself is an evil. Because I was so out of sync with God's authentic design for my life, I was often over-whelmed by that feeling of self-loathing.

Those anxieties have come and gone over the span of forty-plus years but they tend to resurface during times of stress or sickness. When I want to be slender and strong, I find that I am hungry and weak. When I have a calendar full of obligations and a head full of dreams, I am diagnosed with disease. When I want to feel attractive, my skin breaks out and my hair turns gray. When I want to be healthy, the time on the treadmill can feel more like a punishment rather than invigorating, healing exercise.

Judging from the massive profits of both the diet and pharmaceutical industries, I'm confident that I'm not the only one who has been made to feel half-crazy by the disordered messages aimed at our psyches and wallets!

Many of us have come to despise our bodies and, when we pick up a book about health and wellness, we do so with the idea that we are ready to crack down. We are ready to begin again to force into submission the disappointing, wayward figure in the mirror. This, of course, when properly ordered, can be a very Catholic approach to disciplining the unruly flesh! St. Paul says, "I pommel my body and subdue it, lest after preaching to others I myself should be disqualified." (1 Cor 9:27)

However, we tend to misapply the rod, failing to properly identify the source of our failures and the remedy required to make things right again. As illness and disease begin to emerge and impact our aging bodies, the emotional complexity increases. Though we still have the same youthful hopes and dreams, the body is tired...so tired. Sometimes we attempt to correct harmful practices and find that we have neither the motivation nor the stamina to do so. Failures heap upon failures. Where does it end? Unfortunately, it often simply results in more self-loathing, and a passing on of negative messages to the next generation of souls entrusted to our care.

Whether you are male or female, young or old, this message is for you and your children:

Your body is NOT the enemy.

Everything in Sacred Scripture and Sacred Tradition points to the fact that your body is a gift to be treated with dignity and honor because it is a temple of the living God made in His very image. Not only that, but you are deeply loved. *That does not conflict with the need to discipline the flesh but rather complements the mission.* Once we begin to understand the tremendous value and efficacy of orderly, small actions performed with great love, we can begin to break free from the horrible cycles of self-loathing, self-glorification, and self-abuse.

The sins of the flesh are not the flesh itself. Our disordered urges and vices do not define God or his gift. They are a distortion. That St. Paul fought to subdue the unholy inclinations of his body in no way indicates that he was permitted to abuse his body (in fact, we find that the Church condemned the example of Origen). No, the opposite is true: Paul practiced self-discipline in order to dispose himself toward

God's design and holy vision for humanity and to be of service to Christ and to the world.

If you are looking for the latest trend on how to deprive or hammer the body into physical perfection, you will not find it in these pages. Nor will you find a Hollywood diet, fashionable fad, or the latest craze. Rather, our purpose is to ignite a deep love for the gift of our design and to highlight and recommend actions which honor God and His design for us.

In this section, we will examine the most important aspects of that design for our physical well-being:

- Food
- Movement
- Stress-management and Rest
- Environment

FOOD IS NOT THE ENEMY

...For the Church cannot but encourage everything that serves the harmonious development of the human body, rightly considered the masterpiece of the whole of creation. — Pope St. John Paul II

Food is good and beautiful! It is a source of tremendous grace and is designed to be a physical, social, emotional, and healing anchor in our lives. Few would argue with the idea that food is a good reason to give gratitude and praise to the Lord.

The irony is that this source of great joy is simultaneously the cause of much anxiety! We wax eloquent about the beauty of the Catholic table and the importance of the feast in our liturgical year, but when the feasting is over, most of us would still like to fit into our favorite clothes and keep our blood pressure within reasonable limits.

How do we reconcile this tension? I'm not going to say it is easy but I will say that the principle is uncomplicated:

Freedom lies in the act of consistently choosing healing foods rather than harmful foods, one mouthful at a time.

A positive and prudent relationship with food sets the stage for a balanced and affirmative relationship with our bodies. Instead of living a model of binging and deprivation, we have the opportunity to eat for positive, nourishing, and holy reasons.

Some reject the idea that we should limit our enjoyment of eating at all, or that there is any moral value to food. This approach is a denial of God's design which thrives according to His provision, and is a sure path to gluttony. When we put God first and think often of His perfectly-ordered design, we are more inclined to see the simpler side of food and begin to heal our relationship with it and with ourselves.

Food only becomes a complicated enemy when we lose a true understanding of God's provision. We have been duped into believing that the boxes which line the grocery shelves are somehow oriented to our greatest good. They are not! It's time to ask: *What has God designed for our good and how have we distorted it?*

Before getting into some practical information on how to restore your relationship with food and how to allow it to become a conduit of healing, I want to talk more about food as a moral issue and a means to practice virtue in our lives.

THE MORAL QUESTION OF HEALTHY EATING

When I was a young mom with two small children, I attended a local ordination party. It had been an extremely long day for the little ones, and I, as an inexperienced mother, had not prepared well to help my kids through the long liturgy and subsequent gatherings. The invitation to the party was unexpected and my husband and I decided to be spontaneous and accept. The problem was that we had two exhausted, hungry, crying children in the back seat and not even a cracker to give them.

"Will there be food there?" I asked my husband. He didn't know and cell phones weren't common then so we couldn't ask. As an improvised solution, we pulled through a nearby McDonald's and ordered two large fries. The plan was to take the fries to the party so that the kids would have a special snack to distract them from their wearied and hungry state.

It turned out that there was plenty of food there. But we had purchased the fries and the children were eager for the treat, and so we sat them down at an empty table to eat. It never occurred to me to question our decision. Fries were food and food was good! I was unaware of our shortcoming until I heard friends talking behind me...*about* me.

They were ridiculing me for serving our children junk food. They lamented over the fact that parents like me would just give their kids whatever they want, even when there was so much good food available. I was deeply hurt. I wanted to turn and defend myself—explain to them the circumstances and how tired I was and how much I loved my kids. I didn't turn around, mostly because of my embarrassment. I stayed very still, with red face and stinging eyes, convinced that everyone was talking about what a terrible mother I was.

When I talk about the role that food plays in a virtuous life, let me reassure you that I'm not talking about you or shaming you. I know how that feels. I have not forgotten the arrow that was delivered to my heart that day and I pray I never do that to someone else. We live in a complicated world with complicated food, and every instance is not a black or white proposition.

Instead, I offer a discussion of ideas so that we can better pursue our vocation of love toward truth. It is a jumping off place for personal discernment, not a place from which to condemn.

Is healthy eating virtuous? Some people suggest that the idea of virtuous eating somehow equates to punishment and a negative and rigid righteousness. But virtue in the Christian understanding means something else entirely. St. Augustine called it "a good habit consonant with our nature." And virtuous habits can bring us true freedom and joy.

Healthy eating is consistent with good stewardship toward our bodies. It is most certainly virtuous if it is a healthy habit consistent with our purpose and vocation. So no, I don't think I'm holier-than-anyone for eating the way I do. Wholesome nutrition is one way in which I strive towards a virtuous life oriented towards my greatest good.

THE PATH OF JOYFUL EATING

Joy is steady and abiding, like fixed star. Pleasure depends on external circumstances, such as money, food, travel, etc. Joy is independent of them because it comes from a good conscience and love of God.
— Venerable Fulton J. Sheen

Food figures significantly in my story of healing, particularly with regard to the dramatic changes made to the way I purchase, prepare, and eat food. In spite of the fact that my plate is generally full of meat, broccoli, salad, fruit, and other nourishing and delicious staples, my choices still confuse and even bother some people. What is objectively strange about a plate full of meat and vegetables? Nothing at all! It is consistent with Scripture and with what we know about God's provision. It is also just plain good eating!

The only foods (and non-food ingredients) I eliminate are the ones that cause inflammation or that trigger autoimmune disease flares. It's a choice but also a necessity. It's not easy, but simple. Following are the ways that God has used food to bring me joy and restore my life.

. . .

EATING NUTRITIOUS FOOD CHANGED MY LIFE

When I was in my mid-thirties, I was sure that I would be in a wheelchair by the time I was forty. I was in significant pain and I was afraid. No doctors were able to help me and, in desperation, I began a radical elimination diet which changed my life. I cut out all foods that were empty of nutrients, known to cause inflammation and disease, and full of synthetic flavor and color enhancers. I increased and added food that was closest to its natural and most nourishing form. I don't know what my story would have looked like if I hadn't made these decisions, but I remember the despair I felt when I was at my sickest. The inescapable feeling that I had a degenerative joint disease was eventually confirmed through medical diagnosis. Mercifully, in the meantime, and because of the changes I had made, I was no longer dealing with inevitable disability. My body was given another opportunity to heal and be prepared to do His work.

HEALTHY EATING FREED ME FROM BONDAGE TO FOOD

Like so many, I struggled for much of my life with an unhealthy relationship with food. Eating was associated with guilt, regret, and disordered attachments. There was constant dieting and falling off the wagon with intense exercise, not as a good in itself, but as a reaction to poor food choices. Also challenging was the unfortunate relationship between wonderful celebrations and overeating.

When unhealthy options have been stripped away, by choice or necessity, the choices that remain are no food or nourishing food. The dessert table loses power. There is no regret, no internal struggle, no stomach ache, no treadmill punishment. Food is no longer a 'god' but a *good,* which nourishes, satisfies, and fuels my body. My sugar cravings are gone (unless I feed them) and I can eat without emotional dysfunction. It's a tool. A lovely, delicious, God-given tool.

HEALING FOOD BRINGS ME CLOSER TO JESUS

My health issues have been a stripping-down—a dying to my

desires, my preferences, and my expectations. When I realized that being a good steward of my body was going to mean giving up and working hard and paying more, it was a heavy cross that I wasn't sure I could carry.

I no longer see my lifestyle as a loss. As I've learned to cook in new ways, I've found that my restrictions have lifted and expanded. My body craves foods that I used to despise (broccoli comes to mind!) and I have developed a deep appreciation for the miracle of God's design for nutrition. A consequence of that increased awareness is that it is easier to see the love of Jesus in the gifts of the garden. Also easier, in turn, to respond to that love.

When I lose focus on Christ and concentrate instead on my losses, I remember:

If I never eat another cookie in my life, I will still have all that I need for a good and happy life and eternity.

I LEARNED THE VALUE OF FASTING

I'm a Catholic. I'm *supposed* to understand fasting. But prior to my dietary changes, fasting was just a brief respite between binges on pleasurable foods. I knew about fasting but didn't fully understand the physical and spiritual benefits until it became a necessary part of my healing. I learned quickly that many food options in America are not nourishing to the body. Fast food doesn't provide. Party foods almost never do. I was hungry! But when I ate what was presented to me by community and culture, I usually experienced a health setback. Eating out of the house with others became a regular source of anxiety.

It often feels selfish and awkward not to partake in and honor the efforts of good people. I believe this is a reason why so many faithful Christians stop pursuing a healing diet. We mistakenly believe that charity demands we eat what our neighbor serves, even if it conflicts with our health goals. I have heard it said that I am selfish and rude when I decline what is offered, preferring my health needs over the feelings of others. However, honoring my vocation means making myself available for service, which means I am obliged to pursue health if it is within my grasp. That means I need to consider fasting from societal preferences a reasonable option, even when it might offend or confuse others.

Of course, there are ways to demur politely, and sometimes even opportunities to offer a helpful explanation. If people are inclined to take offense, it is an occasion for them to grow in virtue, and I cannot control whether they do that poorly or well.

The biggest obstacles to my choosing to fast from a meal with others are: 1) hunger, and 2) pride. Hunger is a powerful motivator! And the last thing for which I want to be noticed is my eating habits. If there is a mother in the crowd, she will surely inquire about why I have not eaten!

Fasting has been a valuable answer for me. I learned that I don't have to eat all the time. I realized that eating healthy food allows me to go much longer without food than I previously thought possible. I discovered that it is okay to occasionally feel a little uncomfortable gnawing in the belly and to appreciate the company of people over the presence of a meal. I have learned (however imperfectly) to offer up those moments of discomfort to the Lord as a sacrifice and a thanksgiving, and to die to my pride when others don't understand —a powerful lesson in the fruits of detachment. And when the fast is over, I am not as likely to fall back into splurging, but more likely to pursue good stewardship by responsibly caring for my body. No regrets.

In his book, *Eat, Fast, Feast: Heal Your Body While Feeding Your Soul*, Jay W. Richards writes:

Constant grazing and a diet high in sugar and processed carbs is a very recent trend. For millennia, people ate mostly foods that were only lightly processed. They fasted on some days. They ate moderately on most days

—two or three meals without snacks in between. And they feasted just a few days a year. For much of this time, the restraint was a matter of necessity. Later, the pattern became a spiritual practice for every major religion, including Christianity. Our calendar still shows signs of this lost tradition.

Now we eat our fill every day, offering our bloodstreams a constant stream of sugar. Then on holidays ("holy days") we feast—or rather, overeat. Is it any wonder there's a growing epidemic of obesity?

VIRTUE INCLUDES CARE OF THE BODY

Learning how to feed my body in a healthy way has required that I learn about the design of my body and develop a greater appreciation for that gift of design in others. Knowing that God designed my cells to thrive best with optimal nutrition makes eating decisions much easier and even exciting. It helps inspire healthy habits and orients them toward the Creator. I am so grateful that I have the opportunity to participate in the care of creation on this intimate level!

Your journey is as personal as your vocation, and I will not pass judgment over your diet or health choices. If you can eat the way I used to eat and maintain fitness for your vocation, please understand that I am not the accuser! But if you are struggling, I encourage you to explore a different way. One sentiment I have heard repeatedly from people who have radically changed their diets is this:

I didn't know how sick I was until I experienced the feeling of health.

For most of my life, I experienced symptoms that I didn't know were abnormal. When I was ten, it never dawned on me that others were not in constant pain. When I was fifteen, I just figured that daily stomach aches were normal. I wonder how many others are unaware of what it is like to feel truly well. Perhaps God is using this book to nudge you to take a deeper look at the relationship between your vocation and the way you care for your body.

If I have my health for six months or for a lifetime, I will remain grateful for the gift God has given me here-and-now and I will do my best to maintain physical and spiritual habits which glorify Him.

When I fall short, I pray for the grace to restart and keep striving. When I succeed, I pray for the grace to make Him known through the victory.

Now, let's dig into some practical information on the 'why' and 'how' of building a healing relationship with food. Your plate may never look the same as mine, and that is just fine. However, there are some common principles upon which every healing diet rests.

NUTRITION

HEALING THE BODY WITH FOOD

*So often it happens that what began as nourishment to protect our
health ends by becoming a pretext for our pleasures.*
— Pope St. Gregory the Great

It may seem anachronistic, but it is still true that God did not design
the cells of your body to thrive on boxed foods and lattes! Biology tells
us that our bodies need very specific, supportive nutrients in order to
maintain health and grow...and the rest is waste. Can our bodies
handle periodic rubbish? Of course! But what happens when you feed
your body a much larger percentage of damaging non-nutritive waste
than it should regularly manage? The answer to that depends on
factors such as your genetic makeup, the health of your immune
system, your level of toxic exposure, and your overall lifestyle. But it
is only a matter of time before our individual and generational lack of
respect for our physical design starts to compound and cause irre-
versible damage.

While I don't agree that we need to eat only what was available
to the cavemen, I appreciate many aspects of the Paleo approach. I
embrace the idea that it is important to eat real food that hasn't
been stripped of nutrients and enhanced with synthetic ingredients.

It is also helpful to look at history to see where certain things went wrong in order to restore them to the right order. Modern man has become a victim of his own genius and greed, and can benefit from looking more closely at God's original design for food. Unfortunately, the Standard American Diet (SAD) is not concerned with biological law. As a consequence, we live in a first-world country that is plagued by disease, much of which is self-inflicted. This is not very fitting considering the enormous material blessing we possess.

The good news is that the body also has a remarkable ability to heal. If you are like me and have nutritionally abused your own body for most of your life, then it might take a prolonged period of hard work to realize a stage of healing that brings comfort. But every small step is worth it! I've spent the greater part of a decade practicing 'clean eating' (more on that in the next section) with no compelling reason to return to my former habits. I cannot overstate the positive effect that those changes have made in my life.

What we eat, how we eat it, and what we do *not* eat are short-term decisions that may have a long-term impact—whether or not, for instance, our bodies will remain in an inflammatory state (resulting in pain, fatigue, brain fog, autoimmune dysfunction, cancer, eczema, organ damage, etc.), and whether or not certain genetic markers (predisposition to disease) will be expressed.

Did you know?

- Your gut contains as many neurotransmitters as your brain.[1]
- Your gut separates your food into vitamins and minerals.[2]
- Gut health has a direct impact on mental health and is home to the majority of the body's serotonin (a chemical your body produces that, among other functions, contributes to feelings of well-being and happiness).[3]
- Your gut contains three pounds of good and bad bacteria that are balanced to digest, nourish, get rid of toxins, and regulate hormones.[4]

- Many diseases, such as those of the skin and joints, can be traced to dysfunction in the gut.[5]
- Many diseases caused by poor lifestyle (and some symptoms of genetic disease or traumatic injury) can be eliminated or reduced by eating a nutrient-dense, junk-food-free diet and living a healthy lifestyle. Modern medicine is marvelous, but no doctor, surgery, or medication can replace God's plan for normal healing nutrition.

The fundamental truths of the laws of nature & the natural law are unchanging—and so The Sunshine Principle is radically dependable: **the more closely you honor God's design, the better your hope for comprehensive healing.**

If you exercise every day but stuff your body full of garbage, you are setting yourself up for failure. Likewise, if you exercise daily, eliminate junk food, and eat nothing but carrots, you are still setting yourself up for problems. This chapter will focus on a radically simple plan for restoring nutrition to the properly ordered design, and it contains the framework of my personal nutrition plan. When someone asks me how I eat or asks for a recommendation about how I think *they* should consider eating, this is what I tell them.

This basic nutrition plan was developed over years of experience and study in response to my need to reverse severe symptoms of serious chronic illness. It is also consistent with the dietary principles recommended by some of the most successful integrative and functional medicine specialists in the world.

When I walked into my first appointment at a world-renowned integrative medical facility, one of the first things they did was send me to a nutritionist. Her very first recommendation was an anti-inflammatory elimination diet. She told me that many very sick patients get better without medication by committing to dietary changes alone. I looked at the program description and said (not without some self-congratulation), "Everything in this program is what I've already discovered through my own research and intuition. It is changing my life."

TRANSFORMING HEALTH THROUGH NUTRITION

Although dietary transformation is not easy, it is relatively simple. The fundamental components of a healing diet are: **Cut out garbage and increase real nutrition.**

The following simple and practical guidelines can help you prepare for positive change:

1. Cut out junk food
2. Increase whole foods
3. Shop the perimeter
4. Choose packaged foods with fewer non-food ingredients
5. Eat nutritionally dense foods
6. Eat seasonally
7. Embrace the fat
8. Consider careful supplementing
9. Never stop learning

1. CUT OUT JUNK

The trial of going without chemically-enhanced lattes and chocolate chip cookies is a first-world problem. You don't require them. And the responsibilities of your vocation may be calling you to let them go. If you eat junk regularly and are also troubled by IBS, fatigue, diabetes, joint pain, anxiety, brain fog, headaches, etc., then it may be time to start thinking about the stress you've been putting on your body all these years and the investment you want to make for the future. The good news is that *right now* is a great time to begin to make changes—even small ones—regardless of the challenges you face in life.

Below is a list of ingredients to consider eliminating immediately. I will reiterate: **you are not a bad person or necessarily unhealthy for eating these foods. I list them because they are commonly known to interfere with good health and to trigger disease.** I include them here for your consideration and discernment, especially if you are actively seeking healing:

CORN SYRUP. For someone pursuing healing, this should not be used, even in moderation. It has no nutritional value and wreaks havoc on a body. Unfortunately, it is also in almost every food modern Americans eat—from ketchup to canned foods, breads, beer, and medications. It was introduced to the American market in the 1970's (also when obesity rates in the U.S. began to dramatically rise) and is now a pervasive ingredient. It is cheap, sweet, and extremely damaging.[6]

WHEAT/GLUTEN. Wheat is not inherently evil. Our Lord called Himself the Bread of Life and made the use of wheat central to Christianity with the institution of the Eucharist. That's not something we would simply brush aside! However, the way that the majority of flour is now produced is not anything like the bread of the Scriptures. Beginning more than 50 years ago, modern technological changes brought us a soft, decadent, abundant bread. Unfortunately, these changes have also rendered this flour nutritionally empty and it is now a well-known cause of inflammation in the body. Even whole-wheat bread is usually made with enhanced white flour—low on authentic whole grains and high in sugar.

This is a clear distortion of a good which God has ordained for His people. How ironic that wheat, which is not only a symbolic but *substantial* source of life in our Faith, should become so devoid of nourishment! It is another sign that our culture has placed technology and pleasure above the design of God.

Even if you do not struggle with (the increasingly common) celiac disease, non-celiac intolerance, or wheat allergy, you will still benefit from replacing most of your bread and pasta with vegetables and nutritionally dense carbs. By eliminating or reducing this inflammatory food, you will also eliminate a huge source of extra calories and sugars. A growing number of people experience inflammation and stomach upset from wheat or gluten in their diet.[7] Are you one of them? If you are seeking healing, eliminating wheat and gluten for a time might be worth a try. You don't need a diagnosis in order to do what makes you well.

*As an additional note, there are low-gluten Eucharistic host options available for those with gluten sensitivity. And for those who simply cannot (or should not) tolerate any gluten at all, it is perfectly acceptable to receive Jesus only under the species of wine (the Precious Blood). The Church teaches that Our Lord is fully present (Body, Blood, Soul, and Divinity) in both species of bread and wine.

PACKAGED FOODS. There are many exceptions to this but, in a typical grocery store, if a food is packaged, it often needs non-food chemicals to keep it from rotting, breaking, separating, or to enhance its denatured flavor. Added up over the course of a day (or weeks, months, or years), the toxic impact can be significant. It is beyond the scope of this book to discuss large scale, long-term solutions for solving the problem of ethical mass production and storage. However, I do wish to encourage you to make healthy personal choices in the easiest, most affordable way. Cooking with whole fresh foods, whenever possible, will help you do that.

PACKAGED FOODS LABELED 'GLUTEN FREE'. Make no mistake, the majority of packaged "gluten free" food is junk food and nutritionally empty. Just eat real food instead. I have heard the following phrase many times: "I gained weight on a gluten-free diet." That is a common outcome if someone is simply replacing wheat-based empty carbs with different types of empty carbs…and perhaps eating more of them thinking it is health-food.

Another option is to identify companies that produce nutritious, delicious, toxin-free products, packaged for convenience. There are a growing number of small businesses providing wholesome options, including Sweetpotato Awesome, a company owned and operated by fellow-Catholic, Joshua Kingdon, who uses only simple and clean ingredients. I love his food and I agree with his approach:

I noticed that I really didn't feel good when I ate junk. Hence, I just started to avoid those foods. As I began to grow in my faith, I made the connection between mental health and diet and how those two things help one live a holier life.

ARTIFICIAL SWEETENERS. Most sugar substitutes are unhealthy, trigger an insulin response, increase toxicity and risk of disease, promote cravings, and (in numerous studies) have been shown to contribute to weight gain over time in spite of being low in calories.[8] Try using natural sweeteners like pure maple syrup, honey, or fruit instead.

SUGAR. 'All things in moderation' is a traditional formulation passed down by our grandparents, and supposedly a key to good health. But the contemporary idea of moderation and the body's idea of moderation seem to be at significant odds, especially when it comes to sugar! Modern science recognizes that refined sugar is a source of inflammation in the body and that inflammation is a common cause of preventable disease.[9]

More than 100 million Americans have type 2 diabetes or pre-diabetes and about 90-95% of people with diabetes have type 2. Those numbers from the CDC[10] mean that about 30% of the American population is suffering under the burden of preventable lifestyle disease that has a direct relationship to diet. This is further evidence that medical advancements aren't making us healthier—they are often merely managing a runaway culture of disease.

This doesn't mean that we can't ever have sugar, but it does indicate that we ought to reexamine what it means to have a "moderate" amount of sugar. Are we eating like humble and peaceful servants of God? Or are we eating like gluttonous kings who die from diseases of excess?

SODA POP. Finding this on the list should not be a surprise to anyone! Regular soda is terrible for you and, along with other sweetened drinks, is the largest source of added sugar in the average American diet.[11] Diet soda is not necessarily better and a number of studies indicate that they increase cravings and contribute to long-term weight gain.[12] The American Heart Association and American Diabetes Association have recommended that children should not drink beverages with low-calorie sweeteners, citing potential increased risk of diabetes and cardiovascular problems. Eating toxic foods simply because they have fewer calories is an outdated and ineffective way to manage weight and health. Like sugar, soda has become an ill-placed dietary staple instead of a periodic treat.

INFLAMMATORY FOODS. When you ingest something that isn't bioavailable (meaning that the body wasn't designed to consume or digest it) you will often get an inflammatory response. Anytime you trigger an insulin response, you will also get inflammation. Reversing inflammation is an essential step in the care of any disease, disorder, or other physiological affliction. Most doctors are not trained in nutrition science, so it is necessary for patients to be their own advocates and take a common sense approach to nutrition. If you are sick, in pain—or want to avoid being sick or in pain—you should consider eliminating some or all of these ingredients:

Sugar (including hidden sources of sugar), unhealthy oils (soy, corn, canola, sunflower, safflower, palm), fast foods, processed meats, refined carbohydrates, synthetic sweeteners, artificial additives, saturated fats, and trans fats (partially hydrogenated oils which do not naturally occur in foods).

2. INCREASE WHOLE FOODS

The second step I took to transform my health was to increase whole foods. By whole foods, I mean foods that are closest to their original design including fresh foods (raw or cooked) that haven't been significantly altered, processed, or denatured. After cutting out garbage from your diet, it can initially seem difficult to find nutritious replacements. We are used to eating from boxes and bags and have been desensitized to the long list of ingredients on labels. Changing the manner in which we shop for and prepare foods can be a challenge after a lifetime of eating out of boxes.

3. SHOP THE PERIMETER

Most real foods will be found in the produce and refrigerated sections of a grocery store. Avoiding processed, nutrient-deficient foods means eliminating many of the middle aisles. When I first changed my diet, I found grocery shopping extremely discouraging because it seemed that I had to walk past every aisle. Since then, I have learned to broaden my shopping resources and to think outside of the standard American dietary box. Shop fresh. Plant a garden. Find local farms.

Identify whole food co-ops in your city. And if you live in a cold-weather region where fresh food is far more limited and expensive, just do your best in the grocery store. I currently have organic vegetables shipped to me for cheaper than I would pay locally. Get creative. It gets easier.

In addition to shopping the perimeter, you should spend most of your time and money in the produce section! There is no escaping the fact that fruits and vegetables are the most powerful healing foods you can eat and, yet, they tend to be the smallest serving on our plates. Cut out non-nutritive food, replace it with produce, and the results will amaze you.

4. THE FEWER INGREDIENTS ON A LABEL, THE BETTER

If you're buying chicken, you want chicken—not chicken with a lengthy list of hard-to-spell chemicals listed on the label. I once asked to see the packaging from the 'unseasoned chicken breast' at a local "healthy" salad bar. The employee brought me a cardboard box with a large white label featuring a *couple dozen* ingredients! I am not oblivious to the advantage of being able to preserve foods for mass consumption, but it is helpful to remember that inflammatory ingredients often hide where we don't expect them.

If you're buying broccoli, you want broccoli, not broccoli with colorants and preservatives. When buying food in a can or a box, go for the one that has the fewest and most recognizable ingredients. For example, a simple can of kidney beans usually contains some form of sugar. Put back the ones that list corn syrup and other chemicals and keep looking until you find the healthiest, fewest ingredients added to your beans. Choose real sugar over corn syrup. Choose no sugar when it is an option.

5. EAT NUTRITIONALLY DENSE FOODS

Long-term health does not need to count calories but instead, weighs nutrition. The best path to a healthy weight is a body that has the proper amount of fuel when it is needed. If you overeat regularly, calories will add up. However, it is a lot harder to gain extra weight when your second helping is asparagus than if you are doubling up on the lasagna. Make the calories count and your appetite will more likely regulate itself. You will remember what it is like to be truly hungry, with less bloating to cause confusion or guilt. Also, not all whole foods are created equal. If you are short on nutrients (almost all of us are), then you might want to make your pile of dark leafy greens significantly larger than your pile of rice.

7. EAT SEASONALLY

Significant standardization of food has impacted choices and health in first world nations. There are obvious benefits and advantages to nutritional technology which help preserve, transport, and increase the availability of a wide variety of food. But the disadvantage is that this technology also allows us to adhere exclusively to our preferences and, ironically, eat less nutritionally. We don't eat root vegetables in mid-winter because we can still have strawberries! I grew up in Northeast Ohio where the growing season is short, so I've always loved strawberries in winter. But it is worthwhile to eat more of what is seasonal and local.

There is no single perfect healthy diet for all people at all times, even though we have the same basic biological needs. People who live near the ocean have traditionally eaten more fish. Our cold-weather ancestors ate more fat. Our Mediterranean forebears consumed a largely plant-based diet. It is worth a pause to consider that God designed ecosystems, food sources, and medicinal plants to be well-suited to the climate and people of a region. He also designed the human body to be highly adaptable to seasons and circumstances. I'm not saying that you cannot have winter strawberries, but I encourage you to try to incorporate additional seasonal foods into your home in order to vary and increase your overall nutrition and appreciation for real food.

8. EMBRACE THE FAT

It is time to leave the diet fads and pseudo-science of the 1980's behind! Dump the margarine and embrace a moderate amount of the full-fat grass-fed butter. Why? Because margarine is chemically-laden inflammatory food and your brain and body need healthy fats to stay well.[13] Every cell in your body has a biological need for good, healthy fats.

I have noticed that when I eat more healthy fats, my cravings decrease—and that I have more energy, less brain fog, and less trouble with weight gain. When I skimp on the fat, I end up eating more of everything else and struggling with energy. You don't necessarily need to increase the amount of fat that you are eating, just eliminate the synthetic fats and replace them with the good stuff.

Some of the fats to eliminate completely:

- canola (corn) oil
- cottonseed oil
- soybean oil
- hydrogenated oil
- trans fats (found in everything from fried foods, refrigerated dough, frozen meals, crackers, baked goods, and coffee creamer)

Healthier fats to consider adding to your diet:

- Avocados
- Avocado oil
- Coconuts and full fat coconut milk
- Coconut oil
- Olive oil (best raw or at low temperatures) nuts and seeds
- Organic full fat butter/dairy

- Ghee
- Grass fed meats
- Olives
- Wild caught fish
- Dark chocolate (70% or higher)
- Eggs

IMPORTANT NOTE:

These guidelines are designed to meet people in the simplest place for healing, not to offer specific dietary protocols for any individual. There are many different ways to eat and I am not suggesting that I know more about your bodily needs than you do. We have different sensitivities, health concerns, and goals, and some of these foods may not fit in your healing toolbox. For example, I have found that commercial dairy immediately causes an inflammatory response (aka pain) in my body. I also have to restrict certain healthy foods if I am having an autoimmune flare or allergy.

I have done keto, paleo, vegetarian, alkaline, you name it. My dietary approach now has no official name and I will never market it in such a manner. My needs change, my knowledge grows, and I can adapt my diet accordingly. I've also learned that, beyond the basic biological needs of the body and obvious dangers, I do not know the specifics of what is best for you as a unique individual.

9. CONSIDER CAREFUL SUPPLEMENTING

A nourishing diet is more important than any supplement. Pills will not save you from bad food choices. Supplements are typically only necessary when our diet is inadequate. Having said that, the Standard American Diet is woefully inadequate.

I used to believe that supplements were a scam. That was until I hit rock bottom, had blood work done, and corrected severe deficiencies rather quickly with those little pills I'd previously rejected. Countless

years of nutrient deprivation from poor eating, malabsorption, undiagnosed disease, and ignorance left me severely depleted of nutrients.
Unfortunately, I was not able to correct the depletion by eating a
steak and a hearty salad periodically. My age and body neglect have
left me struggling and it has been very helpful to use good supplements to keep my immune system functioning and my energy level
reasonable.

It is important to note that the vitamin and supplement industry is
difficult to monitor. That means that your box store multi-vitamins
could very well contain international sawdust. Independent testing of
over-the-counter supplements has revealed false advertising of
content, as well as contamination by disgusting and even harmful
ingredients.

Do your research. Pay more money for supplements from a
supplier you trust (to the extent you are able). Don't pop a pill just
because it is cheap. We pay exorbitant prices for medications to treat
disease, so why would we skimp on even more important preventa-
tive care?

10. NEVER STOP LEARNING

Some folks may be looking for detailed nutritional blueprints or
elaborate meal plans. There are a myriad of books that provide these
resources. But my intention is to present basic principles and small
steps that anyone can implement. It is far better to begin with a little
action than to delay progress—don't get stuck in "analysis paralysis!"
Your odds of succeeding are greatly improved by picking one thing
and just getting it done.

Your task for today? Pick one thing and 'just do it.' Buy a few extra
vegetables at the grocery store and eat them before they get fuzzy in
the back of the fridge. Replace your lunchtime soda with lemon water.
Use real butter instead of margarine. Try olive oil and vinegar on your
salad instead of the chemical slurry that passes for most of the
popular dressings. Your victories will multiply while you attend to the
details. Great healing will occur in the midst of the hundreds of little
transformations and triumphs that you collect over time. As you make

small changes, continue to learn about your body and the gifts of God's earth—and how they are designed to support each other.

I don't want to close this section without acknowledging again the challenge of making these changes, even on a small scale. We can quickly become discouraged by the intensity of our cravings and the weakness of our will. Please remember that this battle is not simply mental but also physiological. A body that has become accustomed to functioning on a high-sugar, high-inflammatory diet does not easily give up what can be a biological and/or psychological addiction. You are not a miserable failure—it can just be really difficult. When days are demanding and your failure rate seems high, return to gratitude and to the simplest healing action in the moment.

MOVEMENT

HEALING THE BODY WITH EXERCISE

And when Jesus saw her, he called her and said to her, 'Woman, you are freed from your infirmity.' And he laid his hands upon her, and immediately she was made straight, and she praised God.
— Luke 13:12-13

This section is not entitled "Exercise" because that word doesn't fully communicate the goal of healthy movement. Our bodies were not created to exercise only during a brief and specified period of the day, but for healthy and vigorous movement as a lifestyle. The typical modern concept of exercise is the "desperation hour," before (and after) which we practice lousy physical habits throughout the day, expecting an hour of spin class to compensate for an entire day of neglect. This essentially describes a sedentary lifestyle with periodic movement. If that is all we can do, then we should do it. But our bodies are designed to thrive on the regular movement of the joints and muscles throughout the day. That movement lubricates joints, regulates hormones, improves posture, strengthens bones and muscles, and releases endorphins, all of which contribute to a feeling of well-being and support proper immune function.

A holistic and Christ-centered approach to healthy movement

honors God's design for our bodies and makes us fit for service in our vocations. We need a perspective which draws our bodies and our souls closer to our purpose—eternity with Christ—and allows us to most fully respond to His will.

What happens when we don't get the movement we need? Research conclusively shows that a sedentary lifestyle leads to: chronic pain, brain dysfunction, disease, depression, and obesity.[1] The medical professions (mainstream and alternative) are unified in its acknowledgment of this fact.

The dysfunctions that result from the sedentary lifestyle are, in turn, likely to impact our spiritual lives and our relationships with others. Can we rise heroically in any circumstance to become great saints? Of course we can! But to believe that physiological dysfunction doesn't present challenges for the soul is to ignore the reality of our physical human nature. It is possible, for example, for a sedentary lifestyle to contribute to chemical depression. Depression can lead to despair, which has not only devastating social, physical, and emotional consequences, but also spiritual desolation, where it becomes harder to see hope and accept the mercy of Jesus Christ.

It is very easy to compartmentalize "exercise" and dismiss it as inessential or, 'sometimes essential.' We must fiercely defend the well-being of this precious gift of our bodies, not only because our health allows us to serve Him and others, but because we are made in His image.

In full (and ironic) disclosure, I am writing this from my couch because I am not feeling well today. So this is not a clarion call for everyone to an unattainable standard of perfection. I want to encourage and equip you during the difficult days which, for many, come frequently. Even during illness, fatigue, pain, and suffering, it is still possible to fortify wellness! Healing follows a "little way" similar to what St. Therese recommended—one small action at a time oriented towards the goodness of the Creator and His design for us. It is the "little way" of setting down a soda or taking a slow walk around the block. If we need baby steps, then we take baby steps, but the goal must be to keep moving forward.

The goal of Christ-centered fitness is not perfection, but goodness. We will never achieve physical perfection, free of blemish or injury—and we will all eventually succumb to physical decline through old age and death. As in all efforts of the Christian life, we seek holiness above all things, and this demands a proper approach to care of the body and a rightly-ordered perspective on its ultimate purpose.

For ten consecutive years, I experienced a continuous loss of strength and health. I could barely carry a toddler. I couldn't jog across the yard. I couldn't sit in the sunshine without feeling unwell afterward. The struggle to get to a place where I could *begin to begin* has been a fight so constant and multi-faceted that it is difficult to put into words. When you tell me that incorporating physical fitness into your life seems an insurmountable obstacle, I believe you. I have lived it. And it is improbable that this will change overnight simply by an act of the will. But that is where the change begins—one tiny act of the will at a time...compounded into dozens, then hundreds, and on to many thousands. One tiny movement and then another until change is possible.

Is it possible to get stronger during pregnancy? During chronic illness? During a sedentary workday and a taxing schedule? Is it possible to increase endurance, flexibility, and energy when we've got "nothin' in the tank?" Yes! A thousand times yes.

CHANGE IS ABOUT RELATIONSHIP

I awakened this morning tired, as I often am, and prayed an abbreviated morning offering as I stumbled out of bed. I was late to the day and feeling behind again. But instead of rushing out to the kitchen in a panic, I paused and stretched the way that a friend of mine recommends. Rebecca Dussault is an Olympian and a Catholic mom who has taught me practical ways to incorporate my relationship with Christ into the care of my body. She once modeled for me a beautiful, prayerful way of stretching. So, I stopped and stretched and lifted the moment to Christ. My outstretched arms participated in a physiological good, and a simultaneous act of praise. It was a restoration and integration of the proper order of the body and soul.

Ora et labora.

I felt the panic subside.
Grease for the elbows, oil for the soul.
Yes, Jesus...it's all about You after all.

Endorphins kicked in even as I uttered this simple prayer, and I found the courage to go downstairs cheerfully. That has made the difference—shoring up the relationship of body and soul united to Jesus. It is not the act of stretching or exercising that changes everything, but the intentional act of rising, moving, and giving it back to God like the natural movement of the ocean tides. It is a choice to constantly recall ourselves back to His presence in order to combat the persistent tendency to neglect and forget. The relationship is what makes the difference.

Authentic Christ-centered wellness and fitness is about a relationship of love between the Creator and His created, not about trying to chisel the sweets off my hips after overindulging! I've always known that instinctively, but the accountability of kindred souls has been a game-changer. Our shared sisterhood and fellowship continually helps us to restore and refresh each other and, most importantly, our relationship to the Beloved.

EXERCISE IS NOT ABOUT PUNISHMENT

I used to look at exercise as a way of punishing away the extra pounds and potato chips. I now recognize that my body is an instrument of praise. That doesn't mean I am always at the peak of fitness; but it does mean that I have a strong and healthy focal point to which I can confidently return as I progress through the seasons.

A good fitness plan is one that brings me back into the center of my vocation rather than robbing from it, and one that will adapt to life's changes. Whether you are refreshed for your great work by going out to the gym, or just running around the yard with your toddler, the goal should be increasing fitness in order to lead and serve in our area of influence. We may sometimes feel discouraged by or even disgusted with our choices and the shape in which we find ourselves, but we must intentionally and repeatedly reorient toward the most important end.

OBSTACLES TO HEALTHY MOVEMENT

There is already an abundance of well-organized, faith-centered fitness resources that you can explore locally and online. I cannot become your personal fitness trainer, but we can together address common hurdles to fitness. We can put them firmly in their place without giving them an ounce of undeserved power.

The enemy wants you weak and discouraged—too proud, too vain, too stressed to fight. The reality is that you have many physical, mental, and spiritual battles in your future. Your odds of victory are largely dependent upon the small choices you make today and every day. By breaking down objections into manageable pieces, change and healing become possible.

FEAR

Past or present experiences of suffering can make us afraid. Someone who is in agony does not wish to be touched by anything which increases that pain. It is easy to fall into a defensive posture, intended to protect, but ultimately leading to increased dysfunction. A sedentary lifestyle often feels protective because it keeps us from something that is immediately uncomfortable. Sometimes fear of suffering is warranted, but sometimes it stems from a habit of recoiling from *any* discomfort. In either case, the pattern of inactivity invariably leads to further bodily dysfunction and pain and must be broken. There are many ways to pursue healthy movement which may cause some discomfort, but that do not cause actual injury.

Fear of failure. Fear of success. Fear of disappointment that comes with human weakness. Fear of obligations that come with success. It is time to start praying for holy courage needed to take one step forward at a time—past our pride, resistance to discomfort, dismay at the prospect of failure, rejection, and the unknown. This is not easy, nor is it done in one day. But today is a good day to say "Jesus, please grant me the courage to take the next step in spite of my fear. Help me detach from my pride and offer each small movement as a gift of praise to You."

EXPERIENCE OF FAILURE

Fitness professionals know that the biggest contributing factor to a client's future success is their previous experience with exercise. If someone has experienced disheartening patterns of failure, the odds of future failure increase. It stands to reason then, that the biggest contributor to success in our pursuit of health is the ability to change our own mindset—to create new patterns of physical behavior, and begin again without mental baggage that has no purpose other than to discourage.

In a lifelong war against a will that is powerfully disposed toward comfort, we lose many battles. We buy a new planner, water bottle, and fitness club membership and start again. And again. And again. We conclude that which must be true: "I don't have will power." We do not believe we can overcome that part of our character. But it is not true. The difficulty of sustaining challenging effort is a universally shared experience. Failures in this respect are not exclusive to me or to you, so take heart. The practice and mastery of any virtue is like a muscle that must be flexed frequently and with deliberation.

The key to success with fitness is not to win every battle, but to win enough of them to effect positive overall change. And the key to winning consistent battles against the weakness of mind and flesh is to have internal motivation which drives the will to make lasting changes. People often applaud me for my will power. They can't relate to my ability to decline a donut. But the truth is that I have a terribly weak will! But I do have the conviction that I must not give up the effort for health. I owe it to God and I owe it to my family. Instead of putting my weak will to the test by surrounding myself with temptations I may not be able to overcome, I work hard to arrange my life so that I might be strong enough to succeed. In the same way that we have learned to steer clear of sins to which we are disposed, we can avoid those near occasions. This provides something of a shelter for me while I shore up my weak will.

You may have failed in the past. You will experience failures in the future. But if you can, on balance, notch more victories than losses, you will experience some measure of healing.

POOR NUTRITION

If you are eating candy bars or guzzling caffeine by the gallon to keep your energy level up, you are sabotaging your success. Get back to real food and you will see your energy stabilize. Review the previous section on nutrition for more information on how to build a delicious and healing diet.

NUTRIENT DEFICIENCIES

I was shocked to discover that I needed help with this. I thought that I could just push my way through with sheer desire. I was wrong. If you find that you are exhausted even after getting enough rest and eating well, consider having your blood tested and analyzed, and consider targeted supplements.

For example, if you live in a colder climate or don't get out of the house much, consider adding Vitamin D to your diet. Mine was so low at one point that I couldn't remember common words—I was stuttering and struggling to have conversations. I could not even go for a walk without getting fatigued and weepy. My physician prescribed high doses of vitamin D and told me to stop intense exercise until my deficiencies were corrected. After a brief period of supplementing, I felt like a new woman and was able to increase activity.

FATIGUE

Everyone knows that you can only live about three days without water. Did you also know that your need for rest is just as serious? Without sleep, you will begin to hallucinate after only three days, and you would not likely survive much longer than a week.

Restful sleep is absolutely vital to good health, and to having the energy to even consider the pursuit of fitness. To busy moms who haven't had a nap in ten years...I understand. To working parents who do battle in the world every day and then come home and continue to be superheroes...I hear you. Just knowing that a chronic lack of sleep can mimic disease symptoms, mess with your hormones, and cause emotional upheaval can help you feel less crazy when you hit a rough patch. Do what you can. Eat well. Don't drink caffeine or alcohol before bed. Turn off the screens well before hitting the sheets. Pull out some lavender oil. Pray a rosary. Yes, it is okay to fall asleep with the words of a prayer on your lips and heart—in fact, I have always had a fondness for the pious notion that, should you fall asleep while praying the Rosary, your Guardian Angel will finish it for you.

After nine pregnancies and a couple decades of chronic illness, I know there are times when I just need to rest. Eventually however, I will have to try to get up again. One constant theme of my recovery has been:

Rest, but don't quit.

Exercise is not a punishment but a conscious effort to grow stronger and care for the body. That requires respect for all of the body's needs, including the need to recover.

It is common for people (especially women) to struggle with nutrient deficiencies and adrenal fatigue. Runners experiencing this may find that running several miles further depletes them—no endorphin rush or increased energy—nothing but fatigue. Adrenal fatigue is a common obstacle for aging cardio-lovers. It may help to explore new options such as abbreviated strength and conditioning workouts, such as CrossFit, or high intensity interval training (HIIT). There were several years during my battle with chronic illness when extended exercise of any kind would trigger a flare of symptoms. I learned to listen to my body and adjust as needed. As I have healed, the amount of time I can spend running, biking, walking, or playing has increased. But I am still attentive to signs that change is needed.

TIME

There never seem to be enough hours in the day. There's no magic pixie dust for this. We must simply find a way. Be open with others about your needs and say YES when they offer to help. Get creative and be willing to adjust your schedule to look different from the rest of the world. There's no handbook that dictates what your daily planner must look like. Some people incorporate movement into their family schedule and love the community and accountability. Others find the silence and space of a private workout restorative. Better yet, do both. Regardless of what your schedule looks like, it is not selfish to make time to refresh and strengthen your body for long-term service. It is not selfish to treat God's gift with dignity and care.

STRESS

Chronic stress places a tremendous burden on your nervous system and can make exercise recovery difficult or impossible. I address this more fully in the section on Stress Management and Rest. If you are experiencing unreasonable fatigue after exercise, consider poor stress management as a contributing factor.

EXTENDED SICKNESS

There are times when getting out of bed can be overwhelming, let alone figuring out when and what to eat, when to rest, and when to push it. The key is to keep moving even if it's just a little at a time. Be deliberate. Be purposeful.

Imagine that you are "oiling the machine" each time you move something. Your limitations might not permit even a short workout, but it is still important to find a way to keep the joints and muscles active.

I once sat behind a 50-something woman at an NCAA volleyball tournament. She swayed her arms over her head, back and forth like a palm tree, and then stretched them high and low and around, flapping and twisting from her seat. At the time, I chuckled at her "bleacher workout" but have come to appreciate her actions as more time passes. My kids have been warned that I plan to be like that woman as I age. Sometimes you just have to move!

PAIN

Modify! If that pregnant belly gets in the way, choose a different exercise. If sciatica is knocking you down, do an upper body workout from the ground or a chair. If the discomfort you are experiencing is not pain that leads to harm, it's okay to push yourself a little bit. If, on the other hand, you have worrisome pain or other concerns, stop and consult with your physician. If you have preexisting conditions, it is always a good idea to get medical clearance before adopting a new exercise. Use common sense. But, even if you have limitations, find some way to keep moving.

Do you know what people with arthritis are advised to do in spite of their pain? Yes, exercise! Though it may be painful in the moment, the active use of joints and muscles is a healthy and healing action, even with most debilitating painful diseases.[2]

There have been many times in my life when activity with inflamed joints led to joint injury. I have learned over the years how to target and calm that inflammation through diet, supplements, lifestyle, and natural topical treatments. I have also learned to choose exercises which challenge the body but also honor limitations.

...Eliminating the pain symptom is only the first step. Without going to the next one, the muscles will continue to tell the bones to move in ways that violate the body's design...The only product that's worth investing in is a fully functional musculoskeletal system. It's no luxury but a basic necessity that's within everyone's reach. — Pete Egoscue, *Pain Free*

AGE

Our bodies naturally slow down as we age. Injury, illness, and low energy frequently compound to make movement more difficult. However, age is not a reason to stop healthy movement. Aches and pains cause us to slow down. As our joint and muscle flexibility decrease, we accept the decline, and continue to lose function incrementally as we try to protect our bodies. I recommend overcoming this mental limitation so that you can increase function instead of accepting rapid decline. We will not always be young and strong—but we do not have to passively accept avoidable loss of function. If it's been a long time since you've engaged in physical activity, consider hiring a personal trainer who can guide you through appropriate exercise and recovery. Prioritize it as "health care" in your budget.

FITNESS RESOURCES

Can't get to the gym? For twenty-two years of motherhood, I couldn't either! I have become a connoisseur of exercise videos and a collector of small weights, exercise bands, and other fitness doodads. Even if it takes a little out-of-pocket cash, the investment doesn't typically come close to annual or monthly gym membership fees. The internet is a wonderful free resource for workout plans and videos. You don't absolutely need to spend any money to get a great workout, but the right tools can make a big difference. Dumbbells, kettlebells, and exercise bands are my favorite simple tools for strength and flexibility.

I know how to work out at home and managed it successfully for many years but, after experiencing severely diminished strength because of my health problems, I recently joined a reasonably-priced gym with my husband. The importance of being able to work out at my own pace without the constant interruptions of home is something I did not realize I needed. My pace can be slow and my energy quickly depleted by competing distractions, so this new space has been a great help. I also get regular time with my husband, which was often sorely missing during the middle years of motherhood. Even though I am well educated in fitness, I find that having him with me to motivate and encourage me is extremely helpful. If I didn't have gym access, I would be content. I cannot deny, however, that it is a healing luxury for this season, however long it lasts.

A personal trainer or fitness coach can be invaluable to someone who needs help and accountability. In-person training is ideal but can be unaffordable or difficult to schedule with a large family or chronic health considerations. I can personally recommend Rebecca Dussault (FitCatholicMom.com) and Camille Sansouci (InsideOutTraining.org) as exceptional faith-based distance coaches.

When in doubt, go outside and just move your body and breathe the fresh air God created. He planted the trees and flowers for your pleasure and designed them to nourish your mind and body through fragrance and by purifying the air you breathe. He made the sunshine for you, as well as the rain. Walk your bare feet through the sand at the beach and set your eyes on the horizon. He created the world in such a way that we need the trees to survive and to breathe. He considered us in everything, and we should not waste the opportunity to live in that truth by lingering excessively indoors or remaining sedentary.

BED REST

You may not be on prescribed bed rest, but are finding that you have to spend a lot of time sitting or lying down out of necessity. This section applies to anyone who has frequent periods of indispensable inactivity. I see you, my couch-confined brothers and sisters! I've been there, it's rough, and I'm sorry. There are different levels of bed rest. Ask your doctor what you can do and definitely take advantage of whatever latitude you are given. Extended bed rest increases the risk of blood clots and pneumonia,[3] so modified movement as you are able will be an important part of your overall health. If you are immobile for safety reasons, do your research and ask your doctor to find out what you can do...and then do it.

MOTIVATION

"I sometimes wish that I had a clear diagnosis that would keep me motivated to stay on track." Many people have privately confessed this desire to me. They feel just lousy enough to desire a change, but not badly enough to warrant a doctor visit. The truth is that most of us *do* have enough symptoms to be concerned (weight, fatigue, pain, etc.) even without a diagnosis, but we have simply learned to accept a lack of wellness as normal. We have chosen to take up our aches and physical burdens as a semi-permanent cross and keep plodding along because fighting it seems far more difficult than bearing it.

This may be our biggest cultural obstacle. Mainstream culture is unhealthy, and "health nuts" are considered...well...nutty. In Catholic culture, we sometimes put a different spin on it: "It is selfish to focus so much on my own needs. I am busy serving. This is just what I am called to do."

But I'd like to extend an invitation to you—I invite you to dream bigger. Ask the Lord how He wants you to care for the gift of your body. Consider how better health would contribute to your vocation. What crosses do you carry that you don't have to carry? Dream bigger, and allow those visIons to include a greater level of fitness to live out your vocation and Gospel mandate!

Sometimes I take a time-out and quietly lie still. And I visualize. I imagine and recall what it felt like to race with strong legs, or to jump and swim without counting the cost. I remember the feeling of real hunger with no baggage or regrets. I think back on the type of healthy exhaustion that only comes after a day of hard play. I reflect joyfully on the everlasting future when the limitations of this earthly body will pass away. I will dance before the throne of God and I won't stumble. I will sing His praises and never go off key. I dream about tomorrow and what I hope to do. I consider what I might do if I had the energy and strength. How will I serve? How far can I run and stretch?

And then I give thanks. I can't go backward or forward or change my limitations instantly (or perhaps ever). But I can take a moment to remember and to anticipate and be thankful—to let go of things over which I have no control and to examine crosses that I might cast off.

Then I pray...

Sweet Jesus...Thank you for the blessing of this life. For every moment of joy and pain. For the opportunity to stretch and serve and love and follow You. Someday, I hope to dance and sing for You in heaven...with a body that never breaks and a voice that never goes off key. In the meantime, I pray to joyfully give what I have. And to take care of this precious resource for service while I am here. I am Your hands. Your feet. Your conduit of grace for those I meet. In sickness or in health, I will serve with joy.

∾

FINDING PEACE "IN YOUR SKIN"

Nine pregnancies have put my body confidence through a gauntlet of emotions! I confess that most of those years of battling the baby bulge were often spent just trying to hammer my body back into shape without the critical foundation of Christ-centered purpose. It is always nice to fit into my favorite clothes again, but even more satisfying to find a sense of peace in the midst of who I am and who I wish to become. I am gentler with myself now, and tougher at the same time. Merciful but demanding. I am older, but younger at heart. Weak and strong. Failing and flourishing. No longer alarmed by the apparent paradoxes, I have spent the last few years breathing through them like the waves of birth contractions. When birthing my youngest child, I thought, "This is like the pain and joy of my entire life. I'm not afraid today."

Sometimes, the victories in life are that beautifully simple. Thanks be to God!

REST

HEALING THE BODY WITH STRESS MANAGEMENT

The need to involve the senses in interior prayer corresponds to a
requirement of our human nature. We are body and spirit, and we
experience the need to translate our feelings externally. We must pray
with our whole being to give all power possible to our supplication.
— *Catechism of the Catholic Church* §2702

A high-stress lifestyle is, by itself, enough to throw many people into a health crisis.[1] Our bodies are not designed to live in a state of perpetual stress. Rather, we are designed to live in a more balanced condition which alternates between reasonable periods of rest and stress. The balance that we seek is one between the action of the sympathetic nervous system and the parasympathetic nervous system.

The sympathetic nervous system is activated when the body encounters a real or perceived danger or injury. Essentially, it exists to save our lives! It is commonly known as the "fight or flight" response of the body to peril. When this happens, all non-essential functions are halted or slowed so that the body can focus wholly on survival. The heart rate increases so that the heart and muscles are better prepared to run or fight. The liver releases more glucose into the bloodstream. The bronchioles in the lungs are dilated to increase blood oxygenation. The adrenals are stimulated to produce more defensive hormones. Digestion is inhibited to divert energy to other areas of the body, and immune system function is reduced.

These are only a few of the sympathetic nervous system's effects when activated and, as mentioned, are intended to be a temporary state for the body. In semi-permanent doses, this heightened condition will leave you exhausted and sick. When health care professionals say that stress is bad for you, this is what they are talking about!

On the other hand, the parasympathetic nervous system controls your body's ability to relax, calm down, and recover. After a stressful event, it returns the body to a resting state. It replenishes glucose and energy, which were depleted by the sympathetic nervous system, and allows body systems to recover from the stress load. It is vital to long-term health and absolutely necessary to a state of healing.

Unfortunately for modern Americans who live in a constant state of stress, the parasympathetic is slow to counteract the sudden rush of hormones that were released instantly by the sympathetic. It takes time to restore non-essential functions necessary for life. It takes time to heal.

The worst health crisis I have experienced (which preceded my diagnosis of lupus and Lyme), followed on the heels of a two-month period of persistent, elevated stress. I believe that state of unmitigated stress was the trigger for the severe flare. It was also a result of my conscious decision to burn the candle at both ends to meet personal goals and my attempt to abruptly correct all of my failures by sheer exercise of the will.

I'm going to be a good mom, wife, friend, writer, housekeeper, and entrepreneur NOW!

Even though I knew better intellectually, I still viewed my chronic illness as a personal failure and often mistook disease-related fatigue for laziness. I wanted to achieve so much more than my health had allowed me through the years, and I resolved to instantly turn things around by a forced expenditure of effort. Encouraged by a period of good health and energy (achieved by deliberate healing actions), I started getting up well before the children and staying up long after they went to sleep. I reasoned that many saints and secular luminaries slept very little, and rationalized that it must simply be a question of mind over matter. Or perhaps it was supernatural grace, in which case perhaps I could impress God with my initiative and determination and merit those graces! I am not (always) afraid of being uncomfortable and so I made big goals and tried doggedly to pursue them.

In the midst of that stretch, I was also emotionally distraught by specific challenging life events. As a result, I wasn't able to sleep. I ate standing up and used any down time to work instead of rest. When I put the baby down for a nap, I took my phone with me and worked. I figured that if I used every available minute, I would eventually catch up to the rest of the world.

I thought I was being strong and productive but, in hindsight, I can see that I was rather frantic, running on adrenaline, desperately trying to force life and body to suit my desires. In spite of all of the healthy lifestyle changes I had made in prior years, I did not fully understand the importance of managing stress and getting proper rest. The price I paid was high. After two months at this pace, I started to have symptoms that I could not control, some familiar and some new. Over a two-week period, those symptoms went from annoying to severe.

My face became unrecognizable from swelling and my body was undergoing a serious trial. I was afraid and felt closer to death than ever before. What I didn't know was that my lifestyle had seriously compromised my immune system. I didn't know that my immune system was the one thing protecting me from chronic, undiagnosed Lyme disease. I also didn't know that Lyme would prove to be the invisible trigger for my terrible cascade of autoimmune disease.

You may not have Lyme disease, but please DO NOT take your immune health for granted! You have different genetic and environmental predispositions and risks than I—but they may be just as challenging or even more difficult if allowed to express themselves. If your days are a string of stressful events and chronic anxiety, I recommend a complete overhaul of your worldview and taking some time to evaluate and understand your own biology. Your willingness to work hard and to lay everything on the line in service is admirable, but *there is no virtue in driving your body into a state of disease.* It is a greater act of love and humility to get less done, so that you can continue to serve as long as God desires.

THE PROBLEM OF REST

I once met a woman who told me that she has no stress in her life. We were at a class on nutritional healing and we were asked to identify areas in our lives where chronic stress was sneaking in.

"Nope," she said, "I have no stress anywhere. My only child is grown and happy. My husband is wonderful and makes enough money so that I don't have to work. I have wonderful friends with no drama. And I regularly take relaxing vacations."

Wow. Good for her!

My suspicion is, however, that most of us cannot relate to her experience at all! For those of us to do have stress and who daily struggle to find space in our lives to rest, the following suggestions may help:

CHANGE YOUR WORLDVIEW. We need to stop buying into the idea that "more is better" with respect to activity and accomplishments. Americans have a uniquely entrepreneurial and independent spirit and we love the thrill and promised productivity of multitasking. Technology adds to our ability to be fourteen places at once and to be presented with new potential obligations every day. We need to slow down.

Know yourself. Do you have physical symptoms of some kind that are persistent and undiagnosed? Are you on medication for anxiety or depression? Take a good look at your lifestyle and consider whether it matches up with your biological and emotional design. Then slow down until you are living at a rational pace. Easier said than done—but worth it.

15-MINUTE RESET. For many, the harsh reality is that stress is an ever-present bully picking on our minds, bodies, and hearts. Whether we are at work or at home, constant demands leave us feeling like we are an airport terminal in New York City. Never closed. Never quiet. Never at peace.

One helpful stress-busting activity you can incorporate into your day is the "15-Minute Reset." Find a time in the middle of the busy day to deliberately calm down and suspend the hormones that are driven by the sympathetic nervous system. If you can do this multiple times a day, even better! If you can only do it for five minutes before someone spills milk on the piano ... okay then ... five is better than nothing.

First, find the quietest place you can and, if possible, put your feet up. The car is a wonderful option for me since the house is constant noise and perpetual motion. I certainly appreciate a dark, quiet room, but also find that being outside in the midst of God's creation is a great source of refreshment. Just find a place and do your best.

Next, set a timer for fifteen minutes so that you don't have to keep checking your watch or phone. Turn your notifications off or put your phone on airplane mode. Even better, leave your phone somewhere else. Relax every part of your body and silence the mental noise. Do not "empty your mind" like Eastern spirituality recommends but, instead, allow your mind to be filled with the simple and peaceful Presence of Christ. Invite Him in, speak His holy name, and then rest in his peace. This can be meditative prayer that refreshes and renews.

If you can take a nap, consider it a blessing! If for any reason, it doesn't go as tranquilly as you hoped, just laugh and thank God for the opportunity to be alive. There is no sense in getting stressed out by an attempt to reduce stress!

CHANGE THE WAY YOU PRAY. There is a common misconception that good prayer must involve being chatty with God. While we should talk to God throughout our day, our self-absorption can sometimes interfere with God-centered prayer. Prayer is entering into relationship, not recording our worries into a microphone. Just as people in healthy relationships learn to be at peace during quiet times as well as talkative times, so should we pursue healthy silence with God to compliment our vocal prayers.

That said, it is better to come before God imperfectly than not at all. I only offer this suggestion for those who return from prayer as anxious as they entered. This may be because they have only been talking to God about their anxieties and have forgotten to also listen and rest. It is possible to adjust mental prayer to be more fully open to God's healing grace.

The secular world has discovered the healing power of meditation for the body, and science agrees that there is a positive chemical change when some kind of prayer is introduced.[2] Consequently, most naturopaths and functional medicine doctors will recommend some form of prayer or mindfulness routine. Many of the recommendations are not rooted in Christian beliefs (and I exhort you to avoid those) but can easily and most beneficially be replaced by a healthy, holy prayer routine.

The rosary is an under-appreciated and powerful tool for all aspects of healing. It allows us to speak to God in a measured and peaceful way without a thousand thoughts to complicate. Far from being "rote prayer," the simple formula is a rhythmic expression of love that reveals and expands the trust and vulnerability of our relationship to God. Praying as a family or in community is also a way to invest in undistracted, intimate community without significant disruption of schedules. It works beautifully as one form of the 15-minute reset. I am in awe of the way the traditions and wisdom of the Church repeatedly draw us back to health!

I also recommend the book *Prayer for Beginners* by Peter Kreeft, for both beginners and advanced Christians alike. It is a small volume and potentially life-changing.

"When we pray, instead of trying to produce love in our souls toward God, we should be basking in God's love for us. How foolish to stay indoors in the cold, dark little room off the self, trying to turn on the lights and turn up the heat, when we can just go outside into God's

glorious Sonlight and receive his rays! How silly to fuss with artificial
tanning salons and lotions and lights when the Son is out."

FOOD IMPACTS OUR ABILITY TO REST. The way we eat affects the way we feel. The way we feel affects our outlook on life. Our outlook affects our actions. Our actions affect our physical health. Our bodily health affects our experience of everything, including our emotional and spiritual health.

Throughout my twenty-plus years of motherhood, I have struggled with irritability. Indeed, I have sometimes been a crabby mom! There is no excuse for that lack of virtue. There is, however, a partial explanation for some of these behaviors, which run so contrary to my natural desire to be cheerful. This explanation became clear to me after I changed my diet for the first time. I found that my irritability was directly related to how I felt physically. It is difficult to be kind while battling a deep migraine. It can require heroic virtue to be patient when afflicted with unrelenting fatigue. Carrying that heavy load of physical discomfort while also trying to juggle the million balls of motherhood can strain anyone's efforts toward virtue. I learned the slow, hard way that inflammatory foods have a direct impact on my mood and anxiety level. Perhaps similar changes can save you (and your family!) some unnecessary suffering.

Foods that are known to activate the sympathetic nervous system and interfere with rest are caffeinated beverages, sugar, and alcohol.[3] Foods shown to lower sympathetic response include foods high in omega-3 and omega-6 fatty acids, B-vitamins, calcium, magnesium, and zinc;[4] all of which can be found in a nutritionally sound diet. Pay attention to what you eat and, if it makes you feel lousy, consider banishing it.

MODIFY EXERCISE TO COMPLIMENT THE NEED FOR REST. Intense exercise can also stimulate our "fight or flight" hormones, while gentle, regular movement has been shown to decrease that endocrine activity and initiate recovery. The balance is going to be unique for each person—the key is to know your own body and modify exercise level accordingly. I spent years unable to exercise at all because of adrenal fatigue. My body was not able to balance the sympathetic and parasympathetic nervous system activity, and even moderate activity would make me sick for days. I have learned that heavy cardio workouts can overtax my body, but light weight-training does not. Now that my body is in a healthier place and I am better at managing stress, I am able to carefully incorporate more cardio and intensity into my workouts.

Pay attention. Keep moving. Know your body. Don't be afraid to push yourself but be prepared to modify, adjust, and conquer!

ENVIRONMENT

HEALING THE BODY THROUGH LIFESTYLE

It cannot be too often repeated how much the work of the land generates physical and moral health, for nothing does more to brace the system than this beneficent contact with nature which proceeds directly from the hand of the Creator. The land is not a betrayer; it is not subject to the fickleness, the false appearances, the artificial and unhealthy attractions of the grasping city. Its stability, its wise and regular course, the enduring majesty of the rhythm of the seasons are so many reflections of the divine attributes. — Letter of Pope Pius XII

It has become so commonplace to hear about the toxins in our food, air, water, shampoos, and every other item we use that most of us have become desensitized to the message. We are tired and busy and it takes energy and time to sort through the marketing gimmicks, health warnings, and corporate chicanery. We all understand it. We want to do better. We wince when we recognize known (or probable) carcinogens in our personal care or cleaning products and then we buy a "natural" product for twice the price to ease our conscience. If we don't love it or can't afford it, we decide we'd rather take our chances with the seemingly distant possibility of toxin-induced disease than spend the money. We care, but we are surrounded by toxic chemicals. How much impact can we really have anyway?

MY BODY SAID "ENOUGH"

When I was a freshman in high school, I was given a pretty tube of lotion from a popular bath and body shop. It was the middle of winter and my face was dry so, in the middle of the school day, I used some of the sweet smelling lotion on my skin. Within minutes, I looked like a puffy lobster and felt itchy and ill. I learned quickly that the smelly delights of girly life were not for me. I never considered it a "health" issue, but vanity is a powerful motivator for a teenage girl! I learned to steer clear of certain products.

Years later, when I changed my nutrition habits and became a food label reader, I began to make the connection between environment and systemic health. I spent so much energy inspecting my food labels to protect my organs and yet I hadn't been respecting my skin (the largest organ!), my lungs, and everything else affected by these substances. The toxic chemical-sickness connection began to click: *My body hates this stuff. All of it.*

Many of my chronic symptoms started to make more sense. Migraines, respiratory issues, hives, extreme and sudden fatigue—I began to notice patterns of immediate reactions related to products I was using. My eyes were opened. What was I doing? Why was I using products with ingredients that are known to cause cancer and cross the placenta? During my last pregnancy, I learned that tests done on newborn cord blood revealed the presence of over 200 chemicals![1] I began to make changes.

What I didn't know then is that I was born with–get ready for this one–compound heterozygous MTHFR genetic mutations.[2] In simple terms, this means that my body has reduced methylation and difficulty processing and disposing of toxins.[3] I was also unaware that I had Lyme disease and multiple autoimmune diseases including lupus, which is often triggered (and can even be caused) by chemical exposure.[4] The body is not designed to absorb toxic ingredients over a certain threshold. In my case, it was a blessing to be so immediately reactive to some of these poisons because it made my decision to forgo these products an easy one. But please understand that these toxins can also cause disease in otherwise healthy people. Such exposure can precipitate genetic expression of chronic diseases such as cancer, thyroid disorders, autism,[5] and multiple sclerosis.

By the time the average American goes to bed at night, we have come into contact with thousands of toxic chemicals. Before we even step out the door in the morning, we have used them to wash, moisturize our skin, paint our faces, deodorize, spray our hair, perfume our bodies, flavor our coffee, and even eat our breakfast. We spray them all over our lawns for the sake of a certain shade of green grass, where we inhale them and allow our children to play barefoot. It absorbs into our skin, gets inhaled into our lungs, and finds its way into our soil and water. This is the price that we pay to live in suburbia, but is it worth it? Is this really the best way or have we just lost touch with a better way?

People tell me that they are glad they don't have chemical sensitivities like I do, but then they tell me in the next breath about their fatigue and migraines and IBS. They describe their allergies in detail, and lament the eczema and asthma which plague their children. Perhaps these malfunctions of the body are not a flaw in bodily design but a problem with environment.

The root cause of toxic overexposure is rarely known or addressed, and the chemical burden borne by our bodies may only be compounded by the pharmaceuticals we take to mask the symptoms that are caused or exacerbated by that same toxic overload. Talk about a vicious cycle! Making changes in the short term may sound expensive and inconvenient (though I believe this is often overstated). But the long-term expense in medical care is far more costly in time, money, resources, and quality of life. We are, in fact, poisoning ourselves by degrees with the products we use.

You are made in the image and likeness of God. So this is not an alarmist position, but a reasonable objection to the large-scale harm being perpetrated against the crowning glory of God's creation. This harm is opposed to God's design because it damages the very people for whom He suffered and died, and renders people less fit for their mission and life's purpose.

MAKING CHANGES

I know that some of you are going to say: "Look. We live in a toxic world. We can't escape it. I've got things to do. I don't have the time or money to be a control freak about this stuff."

I hear you. In a culture where corporate marketing drives our consumer habits, living simply with healthy ingredients seems to have become a privilege for the wealthy. Bizarre, isn't it? We also live in a culture that is plagued with disease because of our dietary choices, sedentary life-style, and focus on pleasure, convenience, and gluttony. Sometimes, we need to just say...

I don't want to buy in. God made me for more.

So what now? This is a consumer problem. It is about what we use on a daily basis through inattention or necessity, and where we choose to make our purchases. We wear makeup, wash our hair, clean our floors, lotion our legs, apply deodorant, wear perfume, burn candles, and spray air fresheners. We shop and consume constantly. That isn't necessarily a bad thing, unless we fail to align principles of faith to our purchases insofar as we are able.

When some people first become interested in cleaning up their environment and personal care products, they spend a tremendous amount of money replacing their old products with many new prod- ucts. This can cause bank-account-burnout, but it doesn't have to be that way. It is possible to do this frugally, though it may involve some sacrifices. For example, I have found a wonderful makeup that doesn't cause my face to swell. It costs more than the drug store brands so I buy less of it. I also react to many hair products and so my style (even when I get fancy) is simpler. My hair is straight and it mostly stays straight. Some grays are finally showing up and I will likely leave them. It requires some sacrifice but is also quite freeing to detach from so many material needs. "In the world but not of the world" just got a bit easier!

If such personal and meaningful changes were adopted by a large section of society, we might be blessed with a collective healing of our cultural understanding of beauty. I envision a community where gray hair can be beautiful, even on a younger woman, and girls aren't taught to go into debt to maintain "on point" brows and glacially white teeth. Perhaps honoring our body's need to be free from poisons can help direct us to other areas where we need personal and cultural healing. Perhaps it can help us to identify the areas in which our understanding of what is beautiful and true have become disordered.

If you don't think you're ready to make huge lifestyle changes, then consider making just one. Small victories are not failures!

SUMMARY: A SIMPLE PLAN FOR PHYSICAL RESTORATION

- Focus on nutrition. It is the foundation for all health care.
- Consider quality supplements.
- Add healthy movement into your lifestyle.
- Get adequate sleep.
- Learn how to manage stress levels.
- Create a healthy environment by examining the home and personal care products you use.
- Remember that our relationship with food, exercise, environment, and rest are healthiest when they are rooted in a relationship with Christ.

7

HEALING THE MIND

Each of us makes his own weather, determines the color of the skies in the emotional universe which he inhabits. — Venerable Fulton Sheen

---

*W*here is your joy? Where is your happiness? Depression and anxiety are a plague on our society. Is there anyone who doesn't seem to suffer from them? Social media has blown that secret door wide open in recent years to give us a peek into the struggles of others—some of whom we know and even strangers...

The ones who are always smiling.

The ones who seem to have it all together.

The ones with the beautiful children and the supportive spouses.

The ones with the cleanest homes, the best jobs, the active lifestyles, the lavish vacations, the most positive outlook on life.

Yet this social media veneer is as deceiving as it is thin. These are also the people who are sometimes gripped by crippling darkness and anxiety, and who routinely rely on medication, caffeine, alcohol, and various forms of addiction to keep them going every day. Maybe this is even someone you know. Perhaps, maybe, it is you.

A personal trainer once told me about her time coaching middle-aged women at a fitness club. Almost without exception, the women were medicating daily for anxiety or depression. I cannot speak to each individual's health needs and don't wish to try—but is this really the new normal for our culture? Are we so defective that we cannot function without drugs? Rather than assuming that God messed up our design or that most of us require pharmaceuticals to function normally, I must conclude that there must be something wrong with our way of living. To borrow a common phrase from the wellness world:

When a flower doesn't bloom, you fix the environment in which it grows, not the flower.[1]

A LITTLE PATH TO HEALING

Some professionals believe that St. Therese of Lisieux suffered from clinical depression toward the end of her life. This theory is consistent with the biological effect of the oxygen deprivation caused by end-stage tuberculosis. This depressive effect is a chemical reaction that impacts the mind through no fault of the sick person. In spite of that heavy burden, she carried her cross courageously until her final Easter and used her Little Way to stay close to the heart of Jesus. That Little Way rests on the very plain idea that the fastest and surest way to Christ is to do the smallest actions with great love. She lived a hidden but unsophisticated life, finding great victories in the small battles—like fighting off the urge to fall asleep during prayer, and mustering charity toward irritating sisters.

When her disease brought her close to death, she continued to apply this simple approach to her suffering. Many of us carry a similar mental cross but are many years away from our deathbed. We must find a way to keep serving faithfully and with a joy that is deeper than our immediate emotions. Adopting the uncomplicated approach of St. Therese is a reliable way to build a child-like trust and navigate through the burdens and manufactured complexities of modern life.

St. Therese desired a total union with God and found that her losses (for example, her inability to travel as a missionary) ultimately served that Little Way. There was nothing in that purpose or process which would have been aided by a better to-do list, faster cell service, or a broadband internet community. She wrote:

Life is passing, Eternity draws nigh: soon shall we live the very life of God. After having drunk deep at the fount of bitterness, our thirst will be quenched at the very source of all sweetness.[2]

In contrast, modern Christians wear busy, frenetic calendars as badges of honor, as we attempt to exert our way to a sort of Pelagian[3] vision of holiness and success. What is foreign to many of us is the idea that working faster and longer, adding ministries, and doing more of everything may actually be a willful disregard for the gift of our mental health. We consistently violate our basic need for visual tranquility, mental silence, and proper rest, and then are astonished when we become ill, anxious, and depressed.

As more people use medication to manage mental health, there is mounting evidence that the drugs themselves carry high risk for serious side effects. The reality that medications used to counter depression also sometimes contribute to suicidal tendencies. This presents us with a serious cultural dilemma. Where do we turn when the medication isn't the right (or permanent) answer?

We have to look again at God's design and be willing to change everything in order to heal.

When confronted with this truth, many of us feel overwhelmed by the changes we wish we could make, but feel that we cannot. We want to conquer the world for Christ but we do not seem able to resist one piece of cake, or speak a kind word to our spouse when we are grumpy. We will not give up our phones even when the workday is done. We refuse to decline another volunteer activity.

We want the easy way but do not want the Little Way. That is to say that we desire only the solution which will allow us to maintain our preferred pace, our desired lifestyle, and our coveted pleasures. This may mean that we accept a pill as a long-term solution instead of making a radical change. If I were to say to you, "You can be free of (or reduce) your medication if you permanently decrease your activities, reduce your cell phone use by ninety percent, and change your diet," would you do it? That's a lot to contemplate. You don't have to answer yet.

This is not professional assistance for clinical depression or anxiety. Instead I offer simple, reasonable, natural, self-care alternative options. In addition to the professional care that is sometimes necessary, evidence suggests that the following actions, individually or collectively, can have a powerful impact on mental health. One or more of these changes may give someone the healing space to avoid or even eliminate the need for medications altogether:

- Adequate sleep
- Slower lifestyle
- Fewer non-essential obligations
- Good nutrition
- Regular physical activity
- Healthy physical environment
- Healthy friendships
- Strong spiritual life
- Less time on social media
- Supplements
- Time in nature
- Acts of service
- More Vitamin D and sunshine
- Laughter

Undoubtedly, some illness may require at least some medical

intervention to manage. **I am not telling you to stop taking your medication!** But when almost eighty million Americans (including more than half-a-million children under the age of five!)[4] are on prescription psychoactive drugs, it seems vital to point out that this is not fundamentally a problem with God's design but, instead, a troubled culture.

If you suffer under the weight of depression or anxiety, know that you are definitely not alone. You are not an outcast or a horrible failure. You are not broken beyond repair. You may simply need a tune-up. And of course, you need the love and hope of a Savior who knows your suffering. I cannot take your cross away from you, but I am offering an opening for the Holy Spirit to work in your life through an invitation to return to the basics of God's design.

Like The Little Way, The Sunshine Principle seeks the most direct path to God. *The closer we attend to His design, the closer we will come to His healing Presence.*

Research and science agree about the truths that I'm sharing in this book. We are physical beings who have been created to eat, move, love, and be loved. When we have an imbalance in any area of our lives, other areas will be affected. As part of God's plan, we are material and spiritual beings—soul wedded to body...mind intertwined with heart...psychology and physiology. With that in mind, I can direct you with confidence to the pursuit of physical health as a productive place to begin your healing journey.

BEGIN WITH PHYSICAL HEALING

I mentioned earlier that a lack of vitamin D negatively impacted my ability to exercise. It is worth adding here that this simple deficiency also contributed to uncontrollable anxiety and depression. When I finally dragged myself to a functional medicine doctor (because of other symptoms), she discovered that my vitamin D levels were "incompatible with life"—and was only partially joking. It turned out that two weeks of high-dose Vitamin D supplements were enough to significantly decrease many symptoms, and the intense period of isolation and emotional crisis was effectively ended. It was not the first or last time that I was reminded of the strong connection between physical and mental health.

Allison Ricciardi, LMHC is the Founder and President of CatholicTherapists.com and works professionally to help guide people to healing of mind, body, and soul. She shares her thoughts on the integration of mental and physical health:

God created us as both body and spirit ... and an exclusive focus on the mind, emotions, or the soul without deference to the good of the body is a distortion and great disservice. We often see our thinking as somehow ethereal or spiritual in nature and not rooted in physical reality. But this is wrong. As immortal souls are embodied in flesh, our emotions and thoughts express themselves through physical and biochemical processes. Load the physical body with toxins, mess with your hormones, or deprive it of nutrition, and troubling psychological symptoms may manifest. I used to joke that God allowed me to have PMS to help me understand two things: mental illness and demonic possession. This is how strongly a hormonal shift can impact our emotional state.

It can be hard to be happy and peaceful when you don't feel well physically...but even without feeling or being aware of physical ailments, our physical state may be wreaking havoc on our emotional state. More and more research today is showing a definitive connection between gut and digestive health, hormonal imbalances, and toxic load. That gut feeling you may have, that it's not really all in your head, is likely true.

Your thinking, your temperament, your attitude, and your past play a significant role in how you fare emotionally as well. But if you are struggling with bacterial or yeast overgrowth, hormonal imbalances, nutritional deficiencies, food allergies, or toxicity, they can literally be poisoning your attitude and preventing you from changing it. After all, if our emotions are by nature biochemical processes which occur within our bodies, testing to uncover the root causes when they malfunction and then correcting them is imperative to actually resolving them and affecting ultimate emotional healing.

DEPRESSION IS NOT YOUR IDENTITY

My husband has a long-standing practice of not discussing important matters with me after a certain time of night. I have an equally long-standing tendency of trying to do it anyway! He is wise and, in the gentlest way, reminds me that fatigue tends to allow my emotions to overwhelm my reason, and that my perspective will likely change after a good sleep. He is right, and nearly all of the most regrettable words I've ever uttered at him have come long after I should have been sleeping.

The primary symptom that afflicts me when I am fatigued or sick is a loss of hope. As a child (and again in my twenties) I could not discern the difference between the feeling and the reality, and that turmoil easily led to periods of real depression. It was a cascade of physical and chemical responses, compounded by emotional distress. Years later, I still occasionally struggle, but I more easily navigate these obstacles because I understand the process intellectually.

I no longer believe that feelings of anxiety and depression are an innate part of my soul or my natural identity. The intensity of emotional struggle can sometimes feel like a consuming fire. It helps me to reconcile those emotional struggles, not as my defining characteristics, but as occasional companions who insist on walking with me...

Oh, hello depression! What are you doing here today? You've likely come into town on the train with fatigue, over commitment, social media, hormones, my slipping diet, and neglected prayer life. I don't want to walk

with you today. I have things to do. But you are here, we will walk, and I will
pray and work until you leave.

When you are burdened by anxiety and depression, know that
they are not your identity. Consider it rather a combination of chemical events that are a convergence of life choices (made perhaps intentionally or innocently), as well as other factors beyond your control.
Because of that, and in the strength of Christ whose yolk is easy, we
lay claim to the hope of carrying these symptoms with a measure of
peace. We may find that we are even able to eliminate many of them.

THE ESSENTIAL ELEMENT OF HOPE

Studies of human behavior in the midst of tragic events or crisis
indicate that hope is one of the crucial ingredients for predicting
survival. Once a person loses hope, the mind and body respond chemically—immune response decreases, fight-or-flight instinct fades, and
odds of survival diminish significantly.

It is no surprise, then, that a strong faith is a positive indicator of
survival. As Christians, we have that hope, but it can be weakened by
poor health and life circumstances. We must take great care to pray
for and nurture hope within ourselves and to allow the joy of Christ
to permeate our words and our actions, even if we have to "fake it till
we make it." This is the 'pro-life' response to the gift of our lives.

Aaron Kheriaty, author of the book, *The Catholic Guide to Depres-*
sion, speaks to this fundamental human need:

Hope cannot be delivered by a medical prescription. Yet we know it is
essential for mental health. Hope allows us to live today, here, now,
even as it orients us toward the future. Those who survived the Nazi
concentration camps later recalled that death camp prisoners knew
whenever a fellow prisoner had abandoned the last vestiges of hope.
The despair could be seen in his eyes and countenance, in the very
way that he carried himself. In time, the prisoners developed a name
for such people: "the walking dead." Before long, the person who had

lost hope would stop eating or drinking, would come down with a terminal infection, or would struggle and be shot. We cannot live without hope.

Contrary to popular myths about lemmings, suicide is a uniquely human behavior. Man is the only animal that deliberately takes his own life. Suicide is an act that requires rational self-reflection and awareness of one's future. And it is influenced by one's philosophical outlook and social context. Behavioral scientists describe depression as a response to toxic environments. Like the pain a child feels when he places his hand on a burner, depression can be a sign that an environment has become dangerous to the human organism.[5]

Medication cannot be the correct long-term answer to the loss of hope for more than eighty million people—especially since these same medications so often cause harm. Our Lord designed us all for more. If it is His will that we carry the burden of depression (as some of the saints did), then we will endeavor to carry it with grace and a joy deeper than emotion. But if it is not His plan for our lives, let us seek to shed those profane or superfluous sorrows—for His glory and as our living testimony to hope.

A SIMPLE PLAN FOR EMOTIONAL/MENTAL RESTORATION

I propose the following as a rudimentary roadmap for managing emotional healing. Not as a mental health professional, but as a natural health educator who can highlight little ways to honor God's design and facilitate healing.

IF YOU NEED HELP, GET IT. PERIOD.

I'm not a doctor and I don't play one on TV. My role is to help provide you with natural options which do not require a prescription. If you need medication, please take it. This is a practical step you can take in your pursuit of wellness. The quest for natural healing is not some kind of competition to see who is the better hippie! It is all oriented toward our greater good. It is also your obligation to become a researcher, and a passionate advocate and steward of your own care. Pharmaceuticals and medications always come with side effects, and can sometimes even exacerbate illness, inducing severe anxiety and even suicidal thoughts. Advocate for yourself and try to identify someone else who can advocate on your behalf if you are not in a good position to do so.

Professional help does not just mean pharmaceuticals, but can also mean finding a good Christ-centered mental health professional to help guide you through difficult times. There is a growing community of Christ-centered professionals who are filling this much-needed role in the industry.

I believe that the Holy Spirit is very active in these times in calling God's children out of the darkness and despair and into the light. Counseling is one of the vehicles He is using. — Allison Ricciardi, LMHC

HEAL THE BODY

The act of carrying a mountainous burden of sickness and disease, while also trying to balance the rest of life's obligations, is the single most difficult challenge I have ever faced. Now that I know what it is like to feel well, I can quickly identify a recurrence of certain health problems by simply keeping an eye on the barometer of my emotional health. For example, as much as I love cheesecake, I get extremely irritable within an hour of indulging in even a single slice. This is because I have underlying inflammatory disease, which is immediately aggravated by sugar. Prior to understanding my physical problems, I suffered from chronic depression and anxiety. Now that I have abandoned the inflammatory, non-nutritious diet, I feel dramatically different. Life is lighter and clearer. I still suffer emotionally, like everyone does, but I am free in a way I did not know was possible. The erratic emotions I had come to accept as "normal" have been replaced by stability and a significant and enduring peace. So much healing is available to our communities if more people become knowledgeable about how their bodily health impacts their emotions.

The great spiritual director and mental health professional, Fr. Benedict Groeschel, frequently said that "Depression is a physical problem with a psychological effect." His treatment (even before the scientific advancements which came after his time) was always a combination of care of the body and the soul.

PRAY AND DON'T STOP

Even if you just have to call on the Holy Name of Jesus and can do no more, keep at it. Don't be ashamed of the littleness, wildness, desperation, or boldness of your prayer. He loves you.

ASK FOR HELP

Ask for people of faith to pray for you, especially since prayer may be more difficult for you. Confide in people who love you. Tell them about your physical needs and allow them to love you and help you. This can be difficult if you dislike admitting weakness or reaching out for assistance. It can also be difficult if you do not have a supportive community. However, if you are responsible for the well-being of other people, you must set aside pride and find ways to acquire support your own healing.

INCREASE YOUR HAPPY HORMONES

Dopamine, Serotonin, Endorphins, and Oxytocin are chemicals produced by the brain which control the feeling of happiness and help us navigate pain and stress. Some people who suffer from physical or emotional problems will turn to drugs, alcohol, gaming, or pornography to hack into these chemicals—and with devastating effect. Fortunately, there are many healthy ways to deliberately balance and nurture the release of these happy hormones. This will have both short-term benefits and lasting effects upon your overall well-being. Sometimes, just a few of these small actions, repeated over time, can help us turn a healing corner. The following depression and anxiety busters increase happy hormones, decrease cortisol levels, and change our body chemistry to favor healing:

- Laughter
- Exercise and movement
- Physical touch (intimacy with a spouse, therapeutic massage, or simply a hug from a friend)
- Spontaneous or memorized prayer
- Exposure to sunshine
- Speaking positive words
- Listening to beautiful music
- Spending time in nature
- Enjoying good smells (like the outdoors, good food, or essential oils)
- Expressing gratitude
- Accomplishing small tasks and goal setting
- Companionship
- Acts of kindness or generosity to others
- Removing bad habits in speech and action

PURSUE HOLINESS

As I wrote in the Introduction, the enemy of God wants us sick, depressed, oppressed, anxious, numbed, confused, and defeated. Sometimes we forget that we are in the midst of a spiritual battle, and may be lulled into ignoring the presence of the enemy. This makes us sitting ducks for difficulties such as spiritual oppression and acedia. I don't mean that we should spend hours dwelling on the demonic. Rather, we should be fully immersed in Christ, who is our safeguard and our Divine Healer. In order to do that, we must also be able to identify obstacles to Christ and the manifestations and works of the devil. Spiritual fortifications include regular prayer, immersion in the sacramental life of the Church, freedom from habitual mortal sin, an intentional pursuit of virtue and purity, daily readings from Scripture, and a constant effort to grow in knowledge and love of Christ.

Depression is the *inevitable* result of immersion in a life of pornography and other habits which disgrace our minds, souls, and the way that we understand our dignity and the sanctity of others. We need to root out the spirit of the anti-Christ in our thoughts, actions, and relationships. We must allow Christ to permeate our darkest places so that we can heal and flourish.

I would be remiss if I didn't also mention the importance of holy relationships in this struggle. While we are called to reach out with the love of Christ to those in need, our close friends and companions ought to be faithful members of the Body of Christ. If we surround ourselves with those who do not know or love Christ, we will have a much steeper mountain to climb. Besides being a constant temptation to abandon goodness, these relationships also tend to become an emotional (and spiritual) drain. The desire to relax while in the company of those who do not know the Peace of Christ is one of those near occasions of sin. The same can be said of our choice of "companions" through our consumption of music, literature, and videos.

ABANDON THE HABIT OF SELF-FOCUSED SORROW AND PITY

It is not difficult to get locked into habits of negative mental behavior, especially after a period of hardship or loss. This, in turn, may lead to a chain reaction which adversely impacts the chemistry of the body, and even long-term mental and physical health.

Distressing events and situations do not discriminate according to age, and strike both the old and the young. A temptation for youth is to give up in despair at the first sign of difficulty. On the other hand, many of their elders have simply accepted the belief that life is exclusively burdensome and painful. The secular approach seeks to run away from or mask the pain. The Christian solution to these trials is a purposeful life which is well-formed in the virtues and in the habit of service. Our challenge as Christians is to allow a healthy space for sorrow while also adopting practices that communicate freedom and joy to ourselves and to others.

ALLOW YOURSELF TO GRIEVE

You have undoubtedly experienced grief in some capacity. We commonly think of grief as being limited to mourning the death of a loved one, but grief comes in all sorts of packages. Part of the human state is learning to carry the weight of loss. Some of us have lost children...or childhoods. We have lost parents through death or divorce. Others have been abused and neglected, bullied and marginalized. Some have lost innocence, joy, health, hope. Grief is the elephant in the wellness living room, and we shuffle it from conscious thought to stuffed-down-deep anxiety as we try to figure out how to manage the burden.

In the midst of a retreat setting some years ago, my friend and professional grief counselor, Linda Isaiah, offered her incredible insight. Her testimony was integral to helping develop my understanding of grief. When she got up to speak, I didn't think her talk was going to apply to me. I thought that the exclusive goal of healthy grieving was being able to "handle" it and "offer it up" to Jesus and to be united to His suffering—and I was sure that I had done that. As I listened with an open heart and mind, I realized that I was mistaken.

She pointed out that grief is a natural part of life but can become unhealthy, even pathological, in spite of our fervent offering of prayer —and that the goal of healing is to allow it to be transformed by Christ into something fruitful instead of a self-imposed isolation. She shared how cultural mismanagement of emotion is a source of significant pathology, even if it is less noisy and messy. It became clear to me that I had badly mismanaged my own grief.

It was during the middle of her presentation that my own dam of grief broke—like old scar-tissue that burst apart and brought a wave of emotion somewhere between excruciating pain and freedom. I felt the rising of countless years of suppressed grief rush up through my soul and there was nothing I could do about it. It was a movement of the Holy Spirit for which I had prayed and now I was riding out a wave of grace.

Loss upon loss upon loss marched through my psyche and I knew that it was going to find a way out. I had a sleeping baby strapped to my chest with a carrier and didn't quite know what to do, so I ran out of the building and across the parking lot on that chilly spring day to the middle of an empty field. What followed was the most vocal, guttural expression of grief I have ever uttered. I didn't know it was there. I didn't even know I could make those sounds! I didn't realize how much of my life was overshadowed by this persistent sorrow with which I had never properly dealt.

I had spent countless hours of life examining my grief, talking about it, and managing it, but I had never truly mourned. Mourning is not really the same thing as feeling sad. It is not the same thing as "talking it out" or going to counseling. So I gave up my body to that prayer of lament until I was spent. Linda's testimony had given me the permission and the understanding that I didn't know I needed but had still prayed for—and God was waiting for me in the field.

Miraculously, my baby slept through the entire ordeal and I eventually returned to the building, completely broken and ready to be put back together again in the Eucharistic Presence and the sacraments. Since then, I have been consoled many times by the gift of tears without becoming a slave to them. I like to recall the words of St. Augustine in his *Confessions* as he recounted the death of his mother, St. Monica:

"I no longer tried to check my tears but let them flow."

In a turn of events that I would not have predicted, God sent me this gift to knock the fire back into my soul and free me from an oppression of sorrow, to strengthen me in faith, to drive me back to the sacraments that I had been avoiding, and to reach into the depths and expose the most painful places that needed healing. I had been holding onto them so tightly that He had to rip them from me in order to replace them with a restorative sorrow that also permits the light of hope. He is on a search-and-rescue mission for you, too. If you are open, He will find you and free you—God works in mysterious ways!

Please don't give up hope.

RESTORE THE INNOCENCE OF JOYFUL IMAGINATION

It is important to examine the disciplining and cultivation of a healthy Christian imagination in the care of our mental health.

The unadulterated and unfettered imagination of childhood sits contentedly in front of a pile of blocks for hours without anxiety, boredom, or a chip on the shoulder. That innocent creativity simply enjoys the time with peace, delight, and a creative surge. It is the adult imagination which resurrects past hurts and drags invisible fears from the future into the present. Most of us are in need of healing in this area.

Are your bedtime thoughts bound up in fear of failure or grief from losses? Rather than drifting off to sleep happily thinking about God and the future, the modern mind is often besieged by the negativity of our own unworthiness, a catalogue of fears for ourselves or our family members, a film reel of the horrific news of the day, and an oppressive to-do list. Some stumble into the practice of using imagination for unholy purposes—often triggered by a desire to escape from the difficulties of life—and leading to the entertainment of pornographic or adulterous thoughts. Because our imagination can deeply impact our stress levels, our holiness, and our relationships, this is not a small component of health, but a deeply important one.

Some of you are overwhelmed by hopelessness reading that, but please remember:

You are worth saving. You are worth loving. You are worth healing. Please keep fighting. Get angry at the Enemy and do what you have to do to break free. Get help from people you trust. Throw your phone in the ocean. Go find a field and cry out to God for help. Make it a thunderous bellow—desperate, wild, and honest. Think William Wallace in Braveheart. Whatever. Just do it. God made you for holy freedom...not this mental and spiritual prison.

God gave us imagination for His glory and our good. It is worth the effort to restore this powerful gift to its proper place in our lives without making more (or less) of it than is proper. We should also ensure that we have disciplined it and oriented it toward goodness and not harm, for ourselves or others.

As the first irreplaceable step towards recovering an innocence of imagination, I recommend prioritizing a good Confession, where a clean spiritual slate can prepare the mind for healing.

Then try this practical exercise:

Write out a list of cherished things that are beautiful and good. Then choose one (like putting your feet in warm sand at the beach and feeling the warm breeze). During those times when your peace is most disturbed (this happens often at night in bed) specifically ask God to help you recover a healthy vision of the future and His creation. Instead of worrying about a daughter, for example, picture yourself sitting with her peacefully as you laugh and pray together. Try to spend five minutes focusing on one thing that gives you simple delight and restores a holy focus to your thoughts and dreams. Then move into a prayer of petition and gratitude.

It may seem like a childish exercise, but you may find it surprisingly challenging. Do not despair if it is difficult to imagine wholesome things without the interruption of anxious or unholy thoughts. I was alarmed when I lost my ability to do this during a time of great stress and significant overuse of technology. I had to fight hard to restore it through prayer, careful attention, and the placing of deliberate and careful limits on technology. When I slip, I return to basics.

The enemy of God would have us become one-dimensional, depressed, joyless, technology-addicted, ineffective creatures who are disconnected from hope. Even though we may not feel equal to the fight, we must nevertheless engage in it, begging our merciful God for the grace to persevere, and pursuing the small victories which make up the goodness of life.

SUMMARY: A SIMPLE PLAN FOR EMOTIONAL HEALING

- If you need professional help, get it.
- Heal the body.
- Pray and don't stop.
- Ask for help.
- Increase your happy hormones.
- Pursue holiness and immerse yourself in Christ.
- Stop the habit of self-focused sorrow and pity.
- Restore your innocent imagination.
- Allow yourself to grieve.
- Do not give up hope.

8

SPIRITUAL HEALING

The body and soul are so closely united that together they form one person, and hence a malady of one can sometimes be a malady of both.
— St. Thomas More

Several years ago, I experienced the most frightening moment of my life while hurtling down a highway at seventy miles an hour. I was driving our 9,000-pound, 12-passenger, diesel van while belting out Christian worship songs. It was a beautiful day and I was cruising along in the left lane of two-lane traffic with no berm. Without warning, my body froze up. My limbs became heavy and numb and my hands and feet cramped tightly into useless clay spheres.

As a high school athlete, I had the privilege and challenge of running the 400-meter dash. This unforgettable race is an all-out sprint. Typically, after about three-quarters of the way through that scramble-for-the-finish-line, there is an overwhelming feeling of having nothing left to give. But, unless you are going to simply fall over in the middle of the track, you still need to force your body to advance down that last 100 meters to the finish line. Left foot, right foot—just keep the legs moving. My coach used to call it the "rigor mortis stretch." The mind says "GO!" but the legs and arms feel like dead weight.

That's how it was on the highway that day. Suddenly, I was in the midst of the rigor mortis stretch, willing, *commanding* my limbs to function just long enough to guide our colossal family truckster out of harm's way. Except, this time, the stakes were much higher. I was in real trouble. As I raised an arm to turn on my hazards, it required an effort that startled me, even with my athletic experience. Simply pressing the button was out of the question since I couldn't uncurl my fingers. Instead, I had to will my shoulder muscle to *lift*, with an invisible millstone attached, to pick up my entire arm and drop my inoperable wrist on the hazard-light button. I forced my hip to move a leg I couldn't feel. Then I shifted my focus to escape. There was no berm. No exit. Afraid for my children, I begged heaven to send me a way out. Without help, I was certain that we were going to die.

He answered that desperate plea with sixty seconds of grit I didn't know I had and a closed exit surrounded by orange barrels. As I nearly fell out of our van, I knew we had been spared. Breathless, sweating, and shaken, I leaned against the concrete bridge abutment and could feel the ground tremble as the semis flew past. "This is crazy," I thought. "I'm not dead."

Sometimes answered prayers look a lot like closed exits and dirt roads. "Angels" appeared then, disguised as construction workers willing to pull a truck out into highway traffic to keep us safe, and a teenager with a newly-minted driver's license and some divinely-steadied nerves.

I didn't understand at the time that my body was manifesting symptoms of disease, but I thank God for miracles and the wisdom and experience of age. I've driven many miles, broken down in many vehicles, experienced many illnesses, borne significant pain, and had to think through a few crisis situations. This was one of the worst.

Never again do I want to relive that terrifying moment—but I know that God equipped me for it.

After the adventure had played out fully and I was back at home and resting, I experienced a mixture of intense grief and anxiety. That loss of control on the highway presaged physical losses to come. But, at that moment, it was sobering and frightening to think that my body could, at any moment, just shut down.

I have a close relationship with chronic illness, injury, and pain. The suffering that comes with those long-term maladies is real, and the most difficult part is the inability to live fully the life I think I ought to be living. Loss of freedom and control. These infirmities have always been the enemy of joy for me. I have, during times of weakness, unfortunately allowed these thieves to rob me. They have been my silent partner as I strive toward personal excellence—not as a friend—but as an immense and terrible burden. I have named them FAILURE. And they have brought me very low.

In recent years, I have overcome many of those physical limitations, yet they cling to me still, like a pair of ill-fitting jeans. That moment on the highway reminded me that it's not over. It is never over this side of heaven. I felt crushed. Miserable.

It took a long time to work through the fear and disappointment of that incident. But it prepared me in a unique way, body and soul, for the next few years of a different kind of crisis: spiritual crisis.

On the highway, my body froze. I felt almost as if I were watching the drama unfold, forcing my body to cooperate in the most minimal way, and begging the Lord to save me. I recalled that feeling often as I suffered through my crisis of soul, which felt like a terrifying and painful paralysis of the spirit.

A simple prayer was like lifting my numb limb. Impossible. Forced. Frightening. *Where is God? Who is God?*

A life-crisis may be a physical or emotional difficulty which you don't know how to overcome. A spiritual crisis is different, peculiar in its ability to obliterate even your last shred of dignity and desire. A crisis of the soul is characterized by becoming disconnected from God and His purpose and mission for you. Perhaps you are exhausted from fighting off despair, oppressed by acedia, drowning in your own failures and inadequacies, overwhelmed by the monotonous tasks required of you each day. Sometimes we get angry with God and sometimes we have walked away from him entirely. Some have been harmed by those to whom we have entrusted our souls: family, friends, priests, religious, bishops. This is devastating and painful in a way that few can understand.

Each of these kinds of crisis can be tremendously stressful, and they are frequently linked. If you are suffering from a crisis of soul and struggling under the weight of a loss of purpose, joy, and desire, you are not alone. Many of the great saints stood where you stand now, wondering how to find connection and belief again—and wondering how to reach the safety of the berm.

I cannot promise to fix your pain. Suffering in this life is inescapable. But perhaps there is something here which will resonate with you, that will bring you to the doorway of healing and hope. Something to help you hang on until you reach solid ground.

You don't need a lot of strength, just a tenacious and desperate little "yes" to God will do, even if it feels like a kind of dying.

It can be tempting to believe that, if we are just holy enough or try hard enough, we will not be troubled by any affliction. If life were just some extraordinarily long, taxing staircase, we could climb our way to perfection and achieve earthly happiness. The relieving truth is that we are not God, and we are relieved of the burden of being perfect. Sometimes, the best we can do is to hang on and beg for help.

CARE OF THE BODY CAN IMPACT THE SOUL

It is easy to forget that care of the body and the mind is essential in caring for the soul. Frustrated by our limitations, we may perceive that we are failing at holiness, at virtue, at everything. If we were good and holy, then wouldn't we also experience a connection with God and find relief from depression and pain?

An absence of emotion or feeling does not mean that we are disconnected from God or that He is not present to us. This is a common source of spiritual distress which we must set aside. We know Him. He is there, regardless of whether we can see His face, touch the nail-marks in His hands and side, or hear His voice.

At the aforementioned retreat, before dismissing us for a period of "holy leisure," Father Nathan encouraged us to forgo excess chatting and use the time to go for a walk in nature or even take a power nap. He said something like this...

Care of the body is important to a woman's spiritual life. There have been times when women have come to me in distress, seeking help for a spiritual crisis, only to discover that what they really needed was a good night's sleep and the shoulder of a friend to lean on.

It isn't always that simple and he wasn't minimizing real need—but he was acknowledging plainly that our emotions are a chain of chemical events in the body. This chain can be triggered by trauma, happiness, stress, exercise, physical wellbeing, relationships, and even the fragrant breeze on a warm summer day. A meal, restorative sleep, or respite from long illness can make a significant difference in how we see the world, interact with others, develop relationships, pray, see our own worth, approach Almighty God, embrace His love, and accept His forgiveness.

We do not need health or wealth to be loved, to love, to have a vibrant spiritual life, or to attain heaven. Many courageous men and women have lived holy lives without perfect health! But it is also true that afflicted physical and mental states can have a profoundly negative impact on how we view and approach our spiritual lives—and sometimes we need help.

HE DOES NOT LEAVE

My crisis of soul as a young woman led me to the pits of despair and then straight into the arms of Jesus. If I could give you anything, it would be the gift of a loving God. He made you good, beautiful, forgivable, irreplaceable, and eternally lovable. You already possess this gift—and so I offer you instead the reminder that you were created for joy. He desires joy for you. I extend the hope that there is solace from your grief and loneliness. I pass along an invitation to know Him, so that you will never doubt again that you are lovable.

I experienced a second spiritual crisis long after I had become a Christian and had developed a steady and sure relationship with Christ. When everything else fell away and my faith was rocked to the core, Jesus stood in the middle of that wasteland like an immovable force. I could not see anything clearly. I was on that highway again, but this time with a frozen soul. He stood steady, and my hope rested on that one pinpoint of light and truth:

I cannot leave you because I know you, Lord. But nothing else is clear to me and you are going to have to save me—because I am close to lost.

And He does not leave.

Jesus is the answer for spiritual healing. Even if you can't think of a single prayer to say, just call on His name. *Jesus.* It is the only Name at which every knee in heaven and earth must bend. It is powerful medicine for the soul because it is not just another word or a mere spiritual token. It is a summoning of His all-powerful and eternal presence.

Eat a nutritious meal. Drink some water. Take a brisk walk. Kiss your spouse. Call on Jesus.

When you are reeling, find a quiet place to rest your mind and lift up your weary hands and heart. For a brief moment, when you breathe His name, just let the tears fall and give Him your sadness. Give Him everything. **Then give Him permission to begin the healing.**

I once imagined that a healthy life meant high energy, strength, beauty, and endurance. I realize now that I falsely equated youth with health and vitality, and aging with illness and lifelessness (one of the false teachings of our culture). As I age with an autoimmune disease, I don't often feel vibrant, powerful, attractive, or fearless. I often feel tired and shattered. Fortunately, I now measure my health by a different standard—the goodness that I am because He made me, and because He redeems me.

The truly sick are the ones who can find no lasting consolation beyond what the body provides.

I struggle periodically with extreme fatigue as a result of my chronic illness. Sometimes that fatigue, diminished ability, loss of connection, and increased emotional and physical strain causes me to sink to a spiritual low point. I struggle with a burden of sorrow and sometimes even become angry at God. At those times, I return to simple practices of Christ-centered self-care and try to remember the sweet examples of St. Therese of Lisieux and Venerable Fulton Sheen, who gave themselves permission to sleep in the presence of Our Lord.

We can't do it all. Sometimes, we can't do even a little. If the best you have in the moment is to sleep in the arms of Jesus, then sleep and do not worry. Jesus will not leave you.

That I fall asleep so often during meditation, and thanksgiving after Communion, should distress me. Well, I am not distressed. I reflect that little children are equally dear to their parents whether they are asleep or awake; that, in order to perform operations, doctors put their patients to sleep; and finally that "The Lord knows our frame; He remembers that we are but dust". — St. Therese of Lisieux, *The Story of a Soul*

No spiritual master am I, nor have I achieved great spiritual heights. I write, rather, with hope and confidence in Jesus Christ. This is my testimony to His goodness, not my own. I empathize with St. Paul who wrote that he was the worst among sinners. We must all feel that way sometimes. But the goodness of Jesus never disappoints. So let's talk about some practical ways to draw closer to healing our relationship with Him.

∾

THE NECESSITY OF SILENCE

The tumults that are most difficult to contain are still our own interior storms. — Robert Cardinal Sarah, *The Power of Silence*

As I was praying and preparing to write about Spiritual Healing, I was drawn repeatedly to the necessity of silence for all aspects of our well-being. Silence has always been a part of traditional Christian practice for prayer, but even the secular world values its physical and psychological benefits. God's design is evident even to unbelievers, whether they acknowledge His design or not.

Please steer clear of non-Christian methods of fostering silence. First, because they are often presented with a false spiritual message and an "emptying" which is not consonant with Christian thought. Second, because the uniquely Catholic approach is more effective—it offers the deepest possible silence of soul that comes only from the Divine Presence.

There are a great many valuable Catholic spiritual works. For the purposes of this book and simplifying the path of healing, I will focus primarily on the subject of silence because of the great harm caused by the added external and interior "noise" of our digital age. I believe that a return to the practice of interior silence alone could restore mental, spiritual, and physical health to many people. If I could, I would simply replace this chapter with a book called *The Power of Silence* by Cardinal Sarah. Careful attention to his words would completely transform the overall health of our culture:

Silence is not an absence. On the contrary, it is a manifestation of a presence, the most intense of all presences. Pope Benedict states "we live in a society in which every space is filled with projects, activities, and noise. There is often no time to listen or to converse. Dear brothers and sisters, let us not fear to create silence within and outside ourselves if we wish to be able not only to become aware of God's voice but also to make out of the voice of the person beside us the voices of others. Silence is a condition or being present to God, to (neighbor), and to oneself.

PHYSICAL AND EMOTIONAL BENEFITS OF SILENCE

Silence is essential for the health of the mind and the body. The physical benefits are numerous:

- Silence counteracts stress by lowering blood cortisol levels and adrenaline.[1]
- Studies indicate that silence is more relaxing for the body than listening to music.[2] This same effect gives a boost to the immune system and protects against disease, lowers blood pressure, and helps regulate hormone production and the endocrine system.
- Silence interrupts the inflammatory process that triggers disease and poor health and increases circulation in the brain.
- One study found that two hours of silence could actually regenerate new cells in the hippocampus, the area of the brain responsible for emotions, memory, and learning.[3]

The alternative is, unfortunately, the dysfunction with which many of us are living. We are literally silence-starved. Even as we scroll through Instagram looking at beautiful pictures of foliage, steaming coffee cups, and sunsets, we are subjecting our minds to a manner of "noise" which is at odds with the perceived leisure of such scrolling.

SILENCE IS NOT EMPTY

One common misconception of silence—spread largely by Hindu yoga spirituality—is that healing is found in an 'emptying of the mind.'

Even the "yoga lite" workouts that I used to complete by video would frequently remind participants to "empty your mind." Conditioned by years spent in the classroom to be a compliant student, I emptied my mind. I tried, anyway. But I generally failed, as I was regularly distracted by noises from the kids in the next room or thoughts of dinner preparations.

One day, I brought my mind-emptying struggles to a trusted confessor. I said, "Father, no matter what I do, I just can't seem to empty my mind of all thoughts. I try so hard to be a blank page. To just let everything go and think of nothing at all— but I'm failing."

Father replied: "Why are you trying to empty your mind? Stop doing that. When we seek silence, we should not be seeking to be filled with nothing, but with the presence of Jesus Christ. He alone will fill us with holy peace and help us overcome our distractions. When you empty your mind entirely, you open it to nothing and to everything. That can be a great spiritual danger. But if you open it solely to the one who made it for Himself, you are not only finding the true respite and silence you crave, but also a direct path to holiness."

That was the beginning of my departure from yoga and a redirecting of my approach to authentic Christian prayer.

HOLINESS IS IMPOSSIBLE WITHOUT SILENCE

The conundrum of the modern age is that we know we are sinking, yet we insist on having only one hand on the lifeboat so that the other is free for our cell phones. We have music or podcasts in the car, at work, in the shower—and YouTube and social media videos running constantly throughout our days. Even our liturgies can be robbed of silence when well-intentioned music ministers think that active participation in Mass means that every silence should be filled with song.

On one hand, we recognize the danger and actively seek more separation from our lifestyle of noise. On the other, we have become addicts. Several things are clear:

- Immersion in a lifestyle of noise (auditory and visual) negatively impacts physical health.
- Lack of silence harms mental health.
- The noise of technology impacts spiritual health.

Frequent use of cell phone and social media technology influences the formation of the mind and emotions on a chemical and physical level.[4] It also interferes with the ability to maintain and develop interior silence and to pray. If we do not restrict the use of the technology, we may contribute to the malformation of our souls and injure our relationship with Christ. I do not think it is overstating the issue to say that regular use of communication technology has the ability to interfere with our happiness in this world and the next.

If you are a parent, the stakes are even higher. Now you aren't worrying only about your immortal soul, but also the souls of those entrusted to your care. You can compel a child to recite the Hail Mary for a time, but you can't control the noise in their souls during prayer. What you can do is give them (and yourself) better odds for healthy development and the opportunity for silence.

If you or your children are in need of healing in mind, body, or soul, begin with a return to silence. You might have to fight for it and that's okay. Many of you know that separating the child (or ourselves) from the cell phone can be as difficult as removing a limb! *Come, Lord Jesus—restore us with your healing power.*

Gregory Schlueter from MassImpact.us posted his own observations about this modern malady of humanity on social media, and his wisdom is good medicine:

Neuroscientists-technologists are being paid big bucks to addict us. The dealer is in our pockets. They've mapped how pleasure-releasing dopamine design and "hits" work—how they establish and increase addiction to our devices ...

We've become a culture of dopamine junkies. We no longer control our devices. They control us.

God desires our freedom. He desires to break the chains. He wants us to rediscover the vast horizon of genuine, meaningful relationship. He desires that our faculties be rightly ordered and directed...our thoughts, desires, emotions, memories, imaginations.

Attentive prayer-filled availing to grace is the most effective means of attaining a new freedom:

- *Be mindful of the degree of your addiction. How often you check. How you feel when you don't check. Your triggers.*
- *Be mindful of the negative consequences... anxiety, depression, compromising real intimacy, diminished focus, dependency.*
- *Be mindful that you have the power, and that regaining control involves making deliberate decisions to leave the nagging, beckoning "voice" unanswered. You can do it. You will survive. The wave will pass. With each victory, you'll be all the more strengthened, all the more free! You will be transformed from victim to victorious!*

LORD JESUS CHRIST, you have made me for Your indwelling Spirit! Recapture me!

BREATHE. CALL ON JESUS. WAIT.

I once went roller skating with my children and came home with a concussion. Middle age clearly hadn't improved my ability to stay upright on a pair of boots with wheels! When my head made contact with that wall, life changed a bit. I had experienced minor head injuries in the past but this one was different. The pain, fatigue, and confusion were intense and lasted for many weeks. I lost memory and my ability to think into the future. Simple tasks were overwhelming.

Sometimes I would wake at night not knowing where I was. I couldn't place the room or the house, the direction I was facing—nothing. And so

I would lie still in the dark, trying not to panic while I waited for my mind to connect my identity with my surroundings. I knew who I was. I just didn't understand how I fit in with everything else. Once I was driving again, I had the humbling experience of getting lost in my own neighborhood. Lost in my own neighborhood, my own home, my own mind.

I have since healed but I have been reminded periodically of that experience during times of stress. My head aches a little at the site of my concussion, even after the passage of so much time. I feel a familiar sinking and panicky feeling—of knowing that I am alive and present in my home, but disconnected from what is most important to me.

"Breathe. Call on Jesus. Wait."

That had been my formula for navigating every wave of panic during my head injury recovery.

What is real? I am real. I can feel myself breathing and the floor under my feet. And Jesus is real. If all else passes away—if I never recover my mind or my context—He is real. And He reigns. Come, Lord Jesus.

Spiritual healing is like that. Even an act of the will cannot always restore what we seem to be missing. That is when we must make sure that we are following the foundational principles of Christ-centered healing, and then trust and wait for the Divine Healer to apply the cure.

SUMMARY: A SIMPLE PLAN FOR SPIRITUAL HEALING

- Call on the name of Jesus.
- Spend time in the Eucharistic Presence through Adoration and Holy Mass.
- Seek silence. Practice eliminating visual, audio, and mental noise in order to more freely respond to grace.
- Spend time reading the Sacred Scriptures. St. Jerome said that "Ignorance of Scripture is ignorance of Christ." If we want to know Him and to live our lives in his truth and

peace, then we should fall in love with the Bible. Try reading from a physical Bible instead of an app.

- Bodily healing. God designed us to be integrated in mind, body, soul. To care for each aspect of the whole is to honor his design and to bring us the greatest possible health with which to love.

9

THE GIFT OF SUFFERING: WHEN HEALING DOES NOT COME

{The disciples} fell on their faces, and were filled with awe. But Jesus came and touched them, saying, 'Rise, and have no fear.' And when they lifted up their eyes, they saw no one but Jesus only." — Matthew 17:6-8

Behind my sleepy eyelids, I can see the glow of the sun coming through my window. It is morning and I have the sinking feeling that, in just a moment, I will bear the full consequences of yesterday's indulgence.

The feeling is justified.

I try to blink the heaviness away from my eyes but cannot—they are swollen almost shut. My face feels like a plaster mask and a cry of mourning builds up in my throat. I have been here before and the sorrow of recognition hits me like a wave. I have lupus and the sun I basked in the day before was my undoing. Today, I am sick. I manage to hold back the sounds of grief so I won't disturb the tiny blond child sleeping on my shoulder. I gently move my little one so that he is not startled by my distorted appearance when he wakes. There are worse things than a funny-looking mama, but I do not want the added sorrow of a momentary rejection this morning.

I get out of bed and feel the stiffness from the swelling. My joints are badly jarred by the slight impact on the wood floor—feeling like forty years going on one-hundred, and wishing like mad that I could at least have the sweet relief of a good cry. But tear ducts won't work until the swelling goes down, and so my soul cries instead as I touch my face.

I promise God (again) that I won't care what I look like as long as he lets me survive this long enough to mother my kiddos into adulthood. I ask for twenty years (or maybe even a few more). Please.

In the emotion of the moment, I don't know if bargaining with God is okay. I don't know if it works anyway. But I remember the face of the crucified Christ who loves me, and I think it's okay to reach out even if I'm confused. Someone once said that we shouldn't wait to talk to God perfectly or else we will never muster the courage to talk at all. So this morning, He hears a lot of mixed up things from me.

I marvel at how this swollen visage exposes me and reminds me of how childish and unsophisticated I feel. I am nothing but a little girl asking her dad question-after-question and begging for a bit more ice cream.

"Daddy? Why did God make the moon?"

"But why did He make mosquitoes?"

"Why does He let people get hurt?"

"What if we pray harder? Can we stop the bad things?"

Therein lies one of the problems that keeps people so far from the heart of Jesus Christ: *Why, Father, are you letting it hurt so much?* The problem of pain. We don't want the cross. We can't see His love through our pain—can't understand why He would let it hurt so much and what we are supposed to do to move forward.

My inflamed forehead rests on the cool bathroom mirror and I think of life—how much I want to be alive and well—and death—how much I want to someday be fully alive by sharing in Christ's death and resurrection. Some days death terrifies me, and some days it sounds like the relief that I pray for. That desire piggybacks on the emotions of the moment and swells into a deep longing for the Presence of Jesus. It's the desire to feel the warm sunshine on my face but, instead, meeting the surprising sweetness of a rainstorm—finding suffering and consolation in unlikely places, mixed up with tears and joy. This odd space reminds me much of the tension of Good Friday, when we grieve and yet can't suppress the growing joyful anticipation of Easter.

I shuffle downstairs to grab my water, supplements, essential oils (I am an aromatherapist, after all), and to figure out what kind of breakfast will help facilitate a healing day. I poke at my phone until I find Laura Story's song, 'Blessings,' and I press play. I listen and breathe...

What if my greatest disappointments
Or the aching of this life
Is the revealing of a greater thirst
This world can't satisfy?

I thank the Lord over and over again for the gift of illness—and then I put on some praise music and gently dance in a way that doesn't hurt. I can't go out in the sun today because my body doesn't work right and the sun is still somehow my adversary. But someday, I will bask in sunlight forever...

I will not hurt.

I will not be afraid.

I will rest.

I will dance.

I will laugh.

I will rise.

I open my email and see an invitation to come play at the park with some other homeschooling families. The sun is shining, warmly and brightly, and I tell the hostess that I cannot make it today. Maybe next week.

And it will be okay. It's all going to be okay. Rise, and be not afraid.

BECOMING A LOG THAT SINGS

Although nearly anyone can experience some measure of healing from better stewardship of the body, suffering is inevitable and not every wound heals. Sometimes we are blessed with deep healing in one area of our lives but must carry an even heavier cross in another. As Catholics, we understand that Christ and Our Blessed Mother modeled this for us, and that we will never be totally free of suffering in this life. We are invited and called to unite our sufferings to the Cross and to use them to serve others and give glory to God.

Many of us are sick and suffering with crosses of our own making, but also with crosses that have been handed to us by culture, genetics, or grief. I hope to help relieve some of those burdens and also to help change the course for our descendants. However, I know that not everyone will be healed in the specific way they desire, and that all of us will eventually experience pain and death.

The simple elements of this little way of healing in The Sunshine Principle are not designed to eliminate all of your crosses or mold you into the perfect image of health, but to give you basic tools for lifting the weight just a bit—maybe enough to catch your breath and recover hope.

A number of years ago, I sat in the midst of a deeply painful Advent. The world around me bustled and sang and prepared while I was awash in physical distress and mental grief. I did not know how I would ever rise out of the pain but I came across a quote by Fulton Sheen from his *Seven Words of Jesus and Mary* and it changed my understanding:

The tragedy of this world is not so much the pain in it; the tragedy is that so much of it is wasted. It is only when a log is thrown into the fire that it begins to sing. It is only when the thief was thrown into the fire of a cross that he began to find God. It is only in pain that some begin to discover where love is.

Upon reading and reflection, I began to unclench my fists and to relax my defensive interior posture. I was like a mother in labor who, out of fear, fights against the painful contractions of the uterine muscle instead of cooperating with them. There is pain whether we fight it or not, but fighting it makes it more intense and less productive. In an effort to protect myself against more mental, physical, and spiritual pain, I was pummeling the wood of my cross. The result was a deeper grief. The construction of a defensive wall didn't stop the pain, it only interfered with the purifying grace of God. My pain did not disappear or even substantially diminish when I stopped fighting the birth pangs of sanctity—but I discovered the Divine Joy in the fire.

THE GIFT OF SUFFERING

If you really want to love Jesus, first learn to suffer, because suffering teaches you to love. — St. Gemma Galgani

---

I learned a poignant life lesson from a woman who faced a life-threatening illness and was sick for an extended period. She spent many days resting in a porch swing while the kids pressed on, more or less, with their homeschooling. She told me (with a smile) that she never doubted her decision to continue homeschooling even when she was so limited by her illness. She recognized that the most beautiful and fruitful moments of life do not come through absence of suffering but beneath the shadow of the cross and the gaze of Christ. She refused to allow infirmity to limit possibilities and trusted that God had a plan for her illness.

Her kids are all grown now—mature, happy, and good friends—and I've never forgotten what she told me: she successfully and imperfectly mothered from a hammock, and joy grew out of that.

As I trudged through my own early years of chronic illness, I didn't call her. I didn't know what was wrong with me and I thought I was just a failure as a mother, wife, and homeschooler. I figured that, if I only worked a little harder, everything would be better. I imposed a kind of isolation on myself, determined to figure it out on my own. But looking back, I wish I had reached out to her. I know now that she would have understood and that she would have spoken truth to my broken heart. If you don't know someone like that, or aren't quite ready to reach out, I pray that my story and the other stories in this book can be a source of strength and solace for you until you are ready.

Several years ago, God allowed me to partially set down my cross of illness. For the first time, I was able to begin to understand the cross I had been carrying and begin the process of healing—not just my body, but also my careworn mind and soul. I had to learn to forgive myself (this was remarkably difficult), and to parse out some of the confusing details of my life during those years. While I have never doubted for a moment that great-big-Catholic-family-life is a worthwhile journey and blessed by God, I have always harbored doubts about my own role in that beautiful dream.

Why did He make these amazing children and then give them this wildly inadequate mother? I can see now, at least partially, the open secret of the Cross—the stripping down of ego until we rely on nothing but the grace of God.

That is the gift of chronic illness. That, through all the pain and struggle, we are faced with the reality that we are small and inadequate. And that God alone lifts us to glory.

The human family is designed to nurture the bodies, minds, and souls of God's beloved children. We were created to do this and, even when we fall far short of our own goals, that is part of the gift.

God allows our weakness so that the flame of His Love might rise and become a blaze in the heart of the family.

Is the crucifix horrible or beautiful? Is it about dying or rising?

True relief is not an absence of suffering, but the very Presence of Jesus Christ.

My kids love to retell an embarrassing story about me which illustrates these truths. On perhaps a few occasions, I have been upset at one or more children. It was during one of these moments that I was particularly frustrated, and an innocent, inanimate, large toy horse was...

In. My. Way.

I'm not a violent person, but I was unusually angry and assumed that a swift kick to the offending toy would be a harmless outlet for my frustration. Unfortunately, my big toe was firmly on the losing end. It was broken in the encounter and painful for many months.

That toe has never healed completely, but I did learn from the experience. The most obvious lesson was to never, ever kick large toys! But I was permanently changed in more ways than a crooked toe. When I recall that incident, I'm reminded of my sinful anger, my foolishness, my brokenness, and my weakness. And then I remember how God can make all things whole again. Instead of habitually running away from the cross of mercy, we learn to lean into the weight of suffering and find some consolation. It is no longer as frightening because we see that Jesus is so close to us in that moment.

Suffering has been with us since Genesis. C.S. Lewis called it *The Problem of Pain*. It is one of the mysteries upon which our understanding of faith and salvation hangs in the balance. With regard to bodily suffering, *The Catechism of the Catholic Church* (§1501) states:

Illness can lead to anguish, self-absorption, sometimes even despair and revolt against God. It can also make a person more mature, helping him discern in his life what is not essential so that he can turn toward that which is. Very often illness provokes a search for God and a return to him.

Indeed, we see daily examples of suffering souls who choose joy, hope, and service—and also those who choose bitterness and allow the death of hope. *The Catechism* continues:

---

§1505 *Moved by so much suffering, Christ not only allows himself to be touched by the sick, but he makes their miseries his own: "He took our infirmities and bore our diseases." But he did not heal all the sick. His healings were signs of the coming of the Kingdom of God. They announced a more radical healing: the victory over sin and death through his Passover. On the cross Christ took upon himself the whole weight of evil and took away the "sin of the world," of which illness is only a consequence. By his passion and death on the cross Christ has given a new meaning to suffering: it can henceforth configure us to him and unite us with his redemptive Passion.*

Christ is the answer. And so we need to take up our crosses of suffering and healing with equal fervor and devotion, with eyes focused on Jesus and His holy will. It is clear that we should seek and embrace healing, but also accept and welcome our suffering for His sake and the sake of others.

---

§1506 *Christ invites his disciples to follow him by taking up their cross in their turn. By following him they acquire a new outlook on illness and the sick. Jesus associates them with his own life of poverty and service. He makes them share in his ministry of compassion and healing: "So they went out and preached that men should repent. And they cast out many demons, and anointed with oil many that were sick and healed them.*

We are commanded to go out and extend the gift of healing to the world—the Gospel message is, after all, the ultimate gift of healing from sin and death. And we must remember that it has also been extended to us. If we are not healed in this life, let us then fervently seek healing of the soul for eternity.

Servant of God, Elisabeth Leseur, has often been called the 'St. Therese of Lisieux for married women.' Like Therese, she was unable to live out her vocation in a physically active way. Like Therese, she pursued a vibrant intellectual and spiritual life of sacrifice and service. Like Therese, she found her own little way to holiness and taught that simple path to others.

If she is canonized, I suspect that she will become a patroness to those in difficult marriages, those with breast cancer (of which she ultimately died), and those who are suffering from illness or chronic disease.

At a time when I was too sick to read even more than a paragraph or two, I came across my misplaced copy of Leseur's *Diary*. It had somehow found its way to my kitchen and I picked it up with the sole intention of putting it back. However, with the persistent habits of a bibliophile, I began thumbing through the pages and couldn't help but begin reading. On the first page I opened was a letter she had written to a friend whose husband was losing his vision. It was an unexpected consolation to me and I offer it to you:

Dear Friend,

I learn from my sister that your husband has been troubled with bad health this summer, which has perhaps been an even greater trial for you than for him, for the sufferings of those we love are harder to endure than our own. I want to send you all my sympathy and my most affectionate wishes for his complete and quick recovery.

I know what illness is, and can guess what sacrifice it must entail for an active man accustomed to spend his energy freely; but I also know all that suffering means, the fine and mysterious power it possesses, what it obtains and what it accomplishes. After all, our activity (a duty we owe to God and to others) is of little importance, and is exercised only when Providence wishes to make use of it.

And so when Providence prefers to work by means of suffering I think we should not complain too much, for we can then be sure that the work will be done and not mixed up with all the misery of egotism and pride that sometimes spoils so much of our outward activity.

I know by experience that in hours of trial certain graces are obtained for others, which all our efforts had not hitherto obtained. I have thus come to the conclusion that suffering is the higher form of action, the highest expression of the wonderful Communion of Saints, and that in suffering one is sure not to make mistakes (as in action sometimes) —sure, too, to be useful to others and to the great causes that one longs to serve.

All this does not mean that I would not be very happy to see your husband resume his active career; it only means that I am persuaded of the good he now performs in the active and truly fruitful passivity of illness. You will permit and he will pardon this friendly "sermon" from one who has experienced what she speaks of, who has seen Providence gradually withdraw from her every form of activity, leaving her nothing but apparent inertia and who feels that she never did more for God than on the day when to ignorant eyes she did nothing.

If someday I can get about again I will do so; but tell your dear husband again and again that neither of us are now wasting our time.

She closed the letter with loving remarks and assurance of friendship. As I closed the book, I wept. God does not leave us abandoned in our suffering. When my health is poor, my spiritual life can often feel like a desert. But, after having passed through many of those painfully arid periods, I now know intellectually and by faith that God is quietly doing His greatest work. It is my job to hang on for the ride, to give my faithful and simple "yes," to follow a "little way" of virtue—to avoid backsliding into despair or selfishness, and to offer reparation, even when the rest of my body and mind stubbornly refuse to follow. Eventually, He sends the help or consolations we need to show us that we are loved and that He is calling us ever closer to Him. I often wish it was in my time. But His time is perfect. He has been ever faithful.

Be consoled—you don't have to suffer perfectly today. Simply cling passionately with trust and devotion to Our Lord. He is perfect and holds us steady in our weakness while we learn to crawl, walk, and fly. He loves you. Be not afraid.

A CASE FOR PLANT-BASED MEDICINE

And on the banks, on both sides of the river, there will grow all kinds of trees for food. Their leaves will not wither nor their fruit fail, but they will bear fresh fruit every month, because the water for them flows from the sanctuary. Their fruit will be for food, and their leaves for healing.
—Ezekiel 47:12

---

he scent of fresh herbs greeted me as I stepped into the vestibule of my parish church. It was the Feast of the Assumption of Mary. The smell of dill, rosemary, oregano, and basil filled the room and awakened a memory of my grandfather's garden where I used to eat sun-warmed tomatoes straight off the vines. For centuries, Catholics have celebrated this great feast of Mary with a traditional blessing of herbs, fruits, and flowers, but this was my first encounter.

My European friends tell me that the practice is still quite common in their countries. Women gather herbs in the days preceding the feast and tie them in bunches for the blessing. Following Mass, every family receives a bundle of blessed herbs to take home. In my own small American parish in the city, one woman lovingly took on this task.

As I listened to the words of the blessing, my eyes filled with grateful tears. My health struggles have brought me to a deep appreciation for the gifts of God's earth and plant-based medicine. And, in the enduring words of the Church, I encountered the wisdom I had accidentally (re)discovered on my journey.

God has always provided. He has designed the earth with consideration for every need. When He created these tools of healing, He was thinking of me.

A few drops of holy water splashed on my nose and Father's voice rang in my ears...

Almighty, everlasting God, who by Thy Word hast created out of nothing heaven, earth, sea, visible and invisible things; who hast commanded the earth to bring forth herbs and trees for the use of men and animals...and who hast granted out of Thine unspeakable mercy for these to serve not only as for the living, but as medicine for sick bodies: with mind and mouth we humbly implore Thee to bless with Thy clemency these herbs and fruits of various kinds, and to pour forth upon their natural power already given by Thee the grace of Thy new blessing; that when used by men and beasts who apply them in Thy name, they may provide protection against all disease and adversity. Through our Lord Jesus Christ. Amen. [1]

The Church is not an edifice of stone and brick, but a living temple, a Mystical Body, built of flesh and bone. To the greater glory of God, she is a people baptized by water and fire, guided by the Spirit, and fortified by the plants and animals which inhabit the earth. There is no more fully integrated faith than Catholicism. It is, after all, the Faith in Him—and given to us by Him—Who created heaven and earth. But we do sometimes forget.

TRUTH IN NATURE

Modern medicine likes to boast that 'science improves upon nature.' It is more correct to say that we are learning to cooperate with God's perfect design in nature—and we are always discovering more of His perfection in the natural world. It may seem a matter of semantics to some, but the danger of this imprecise language is that we put ourselves at odds with God's purpose and elevate our role to one of equality with God. We were created to love Him, to receive His gifts, and to cooperate with His perfect plan for our happiness. It is not so much a proof of man's ingenuity as it is of God's magnificence.

G. K. Chesterton wrote that, "All science, even the divine science, is a sublime detective story. Only it is not set to detect why a man is dead; but the darker secret of why he is alive."

Science gives us insight into the why and the how of what people have known throughout Salvation History. This is not just a story of what things are, but of who we are in relation to God. Our responsibility is to use that information carefully and reverently so that we can grow closer to God and his healing grace.

Name something good that didn't originate somehow from God's creation. You cannot do it! And that is the simplest way to dispel the notion that natural remedies are bizarre or are incongruent with healthy living. The idea that our most effective healing methods somehow exist outside a natural context is, *prima facie,* ridiculous. And the assertion that science and natural health care are at odds is even more absurd.

A week doesn't go by that I don't see another meme or social media comment claiming that plant-based medicines belong to the New Age. I will discredit that canard more fully in Chapter 11, but here is the undiluted truth: the oil extracted from a peppermint leaf is no more evil than the juice squeezed from an orange. To argue otherwise is silliness. To proliferate such nonsense is simply irresponsible at best and, perhaps, quite wicked indeed.

Plant-based medicine has been with us since creation and was used as the primary tool of physicians until recent history. In addition to recognizing that our pharmaceutical model is not the panacea that everyone has hoped for, modern science is now rediscovering the gifts of the earth through research and study. The "new" emergence of alternative and natural medicines is simply a rediscovery of the original gift, lost over time. The fact that pharmaceutical companies cannot patent or profit from common medicinal plants is worth noting as we explore health care options. The sheer force that these companies can bring to bear in pushing their own research and products for profit and, conversely, suppressing facts and commodities that might harm their bottom line is almost unbelievable.

Dr. Bill Rawls, a physician and specialist in chronic illness, in his book *Unlocking Lyme*, writes:

> Because of science, it is now possible to evaluate the medicinal effects of specific biochemical substances found in herbs. When both tradition and science are considered, we know more about herbs than any other source of healing on the planet.[2]

He then lists the broad range of properties provided by plant biochemistry. These benefits, which are common to herbs, include: antimicrobial, antiviral, anti fungal, anti-inflammatory, immune modulation, anti-mutagenic (cancer), antioxidant, hormone-balancing, energizing, calming, detoxifying, and cellular support.

Most people who take elderberry syrup, garlic cloves, honey, and tea for sickness probably don't consider themselves unusual, or even practitioners of natural medicine. They are simply doing what makes sense and what popular culture has discovered is beneficial to the body. But, because we have largely lost our cultural knowledge of herbal remedies, it is not practical for each family to become instantly adept at herbal medicine. Furthermore, such herbal medicines are often relegated to the realm of the eccentric or, as noted above, even the occult.

It would be wonderful if families could once again take up natural healing arts in the home. Our fast-paced culture might seem at odds with old-fashioned methods and, in some respects, it is. Fortunately, there are plenty of opportunities to implement the advances of that culture in ways that are beneficial. For instance, the advent of internet technology, Wi-Fi, and easy access to education, all but eliminate the necessity of becoming an expert in plants and herbal remedies. In other words, you can enjoy the benefits of plant-based medicine without becoming an herbalist.

WHAT'S IN YOUR MEDICINE CABINET?

Prior to my health crisis, our medicine cabinet was filled with bottles of synthetic medications and products, all designed to mask symptoms of discomfort or override the body's natural functions. But, as I became sick with chronic symptoms, I was unable to take many of these medications without negative side effects. I didn't realize at the time how damaging regular use of these drugs can be, but I was learning through experience that my body was not processing them well at all.

As my options became more limited, I learned more about natural medicine and, specifically, about the restorative abilities of plants. They are so absolutely and marvelously consistent with our Christian belief in the creative, loving, generous God of Genesis! I felt more than a little silly for having rejected these options out of turn for so long.

Pharmaceutical or over-the-counter drugs are no longer my primary resource. I am learning to be attentive in other ways to the needs of my body. I have also learned to accept a bit of discomfort without reaching for any remedy at all. It is difficult to break out of the habit of seeking instant relief from every ache or pain when pills are so readily available. But a shift away from the expectation that life should be absolutely pain-free is helpful in many ways, and so my adjusted perspective asks:

- First, can I do without?

- Second, what is the most biologically healthy option?

- Third, if I must take a pharmaceutical, what are the known side effects and alternatives?

- Fourth, what is the smallest measure I can take for relief?

One of the most common questions I field is: "Why change what's working if I like my medications?"

We are so blessed to have the benefits of modern medicines when we need them, but there are some objective reasons why pharmaceutical and over-the-counter medications should be used sparingly and only when truly necessary. They are a blessing when we require an intervention that a simpler, natural remedy can't provide. But they can also become a terrible burden, giving us a new set of sufferings in exchange for the old. These are typically called "side effects." Virtually all pharmaceuticals have side effects. Some of these are listed on the packaging. Other side effects—and this is extremely important to note —are unknown even to the researchers who formulated the product or the physicians who prescribe it. We must decide whether the need for the medication is greater than the potential harm.

Recently, I met a combat veteran who was looking for natural pain management options. He lives with daily, debilitating chronic pain but was no longer able to take acetaminophen, which he described as "the only thing that helps with the pain." Why did he stop? "Doctor's orders." Regular prolonged use of this ubiquitous drug had permanently damaged his liver, and he is now battling liver disease in addition to chronic pain. He admits that he took doses that were too high because he was trying to avoid the stronger, more addictive (and toxic) opiates.

Perhaps he may not have accepted alternative options decades earlier when he was a young, wounded soldier. He may not have welcomed them as a middle-aged husband and father. He may even have had trouble accepting them as an elderly grandfather who is out of other options. But he was never offered natural or non-pharmaceutical options by those who were charged with his care. I believe that last fact indicates a serious cultural and ethical problem for the practitioners of modern medicine.

Why should pharmaceuticals be a last resort for our health care? Erica Lichter (a Catholic friend, trained biologist, and Registered Nurse), explains why synthetic drugs will always cause side effects in the human body:

When pharmaceuticals are being developed in a lab, a pool of elements and other aiding substances are combined to create new three-dimensional molecules. When the new molecules are formed, the three-dimensional mirror images, or enantiomers, are also formed. The first molecule has the desired effect because its structure locks onto a chemical pathway in the body it was intended to aid or block. However, the enantiomers, being mirror images, are not the correct shape to do this, and they cause other problems in the body. It is the enantiomers that cause the side effects of pharmaceutical drugs.

In other words, synthetic drugs are not biologically friendly, and stress on the body is unavoidable. Although sometimes necessary, they should not be the normal model of health care. So let's talk plants, Catholicism, and affordable natural health care.

HERBS, ESSENTIAL OILS, AND PLANTS ...OH MY!

In addition to using plant-based medicine as my primary form of health care as a consumer, I'm also a Certified Aromatherapist. But, prior to my health crisis, I wanted nothing to do with natural medicine. In fact, the first time a friend suggested dietary changes for my chronic illness, I brushed her off. When another friend recommended herbal teas, I gave obligatory nods but rolled my internal eyes. And, when yet another friend tried to tell me about essential oils from plants, I scoffed. She might as well have told me that she was using crystals to heal her broken aura while burning sage smudge sticks for the shaman! My head nodded politely but I was probably thinking about dinner...or wallpaper...or something.

My experience of "natural" healing had primarily been from my exposure to New Age practices. When I walked away from that environment to embrace my Catholic faith, I purposely turned away from everything that I associated with the New Age stereotype. I banished the patchouli incense, yoga practices, and beliefs in reincarnation. I wanted none of it!

I needed that distance. I needed clarity and time for discernment. But ultimately, I discovered that I had thrown the proverbial baby out with the bathwater. Does that mean that I embrace even a single tenet or trapping of the New Age or occult natural healing movement? Absolutely not! To borrow a phrase from our Baptismal Promises, I reject the New Age and all of its works and all its empty promises. I also now more clearly understand that the natural world, created by God, belongs to Him first and foremost—and that I am now seeing things rightly ordered.

Just because the New-Agers understand some portion of the truth of natural medicines and use it in their pagan practices in no way indicates that it belongs to their idolatrous belief system. If this were true, then we ought to abandon the use of fireworks in our Independence Day celebrations, because they are also used by Communist regimes around the world to commemorate their wicked victories. If something is good, true, and beautiful—like God's created natural means for healing—it cannot also be theosophist or occultist. I embrace that which is wholesome and designed to support us in our vocation and in the service of God and others.

Recall the underlying principle of this book—God has arranged everything in the universe in consideration of everything else. And the greatest potential for healing presents itself when we align our actions with God's natural, biological, and spiritual law.

Yes, I reject the Tarot cards, the Hindu yoga, and the spiritual practices in conflict with a Christian worldview. I am inquisitive, and sometimes even overly-skeptical. I have baggage from my past that exacerbates that tendency, especially with respect to anything that others insist on trying to connect to New Age spiritualism. At this point in my life it strikes me as almost comical, but coming to terms with plants as medicine was as arduous as climbing a mountain.

The science finally convinced me, since the suspension of reason was not required. And, like the central theme of Pope St. John Paul II's, *Fides et Ratio*, science is not opposed to faith. Rather, the two are in a complete and even *necessary* harmony. That is to say, the science of plant-based medicine is perfectly aligned with Sacred Scripture, Church teaching, and Salvation History. We recognize experientially that the natural world provides real solutions to illness and disease. We love the smells of nature and we buy the products that feature them, not even consciously aware that those smells impact our brain chemistry and our overall health. We walk in beautiful places because we instinctively appreciate that it is good for the mind, body, and soul. We breathe it in, feel it on our skin, and bring it into our homes. We slather stuff all over our bodies until we smell like walking orchards and flower gardens. Whole industries have grown out of our desire to be fragrant like things of the earth. We crave it. We literally salivate over the smell of dinner cooking. Boiling cinnamon and cloves makes us feel festive and happy, like it's Christmastime. We make our own elderberry syrup when flu season hits. Extra garlic cloves in the chicken soup help to fight off a cold. And here is the wonderful truth behind all of those instinctive impulses and traditional practices we learned from our great-grandparents:

The scientific data supports those natural inclinations. These gifts of creation were made for our health and happiness.

Just what does the science say? Oregano has anti-bacterial, anti-fungal properties woven into its chemistry. Thyme, cinnamon, and clove are among many others with similar properties.[3] Clinical studies show that frankincense oil has the ability to penetrate the blood/brain barrier and calm brain inflammation in cancer patients following radiation therapy.[4] The oil from a citrus peel has antioxidant properties and the smell protects against depressive feelings by stimulating the emotional center of the brain.[5] Peppermint supports respiratory health.[6]

All of these benefits (and more) aren't restricted to the sterile environment of a science lab, but are available to anyone with access to these potent plants. They are extraordinary tools, and choosing not to explore or utilize them prevents us from fully enjoying the expansive blessing of God's created world.

WHAT ARE HERBS AND ESSENTIAL OILS?

Herbs and spices are fresh or dried plants that are used for specific medicinal, aromatic, or culinary properties. *Essential oils* are simply the pure oils pressed or distilled from those same plants, with similar (but more concentrated) God-given chemical benefits. The molecular structure of plants allows them unique access to our bodies, at a cellular level. This is true whether we are eating them, applying them topically, or simply smelling them.

There's nothing strange, scary, or unexpected about the fact that God's supreme intelligence and benevolence is made manifest throughout all of creation—and for the benefit of those whom He loves so dearly that He gave His only begotten Son!

As traditional herbal medicine has fallen out of practice in modernized nations where pharmaceutical drugs are preferred, we have lost our collective memory of their important role in our health care. One recent technological innovation which is helping us to restore that gap is the significant production of essential oils. This plant-focused method combines the efficacy of traditional herbal medicine with the technology of our time. It allows us to press or distill oils from different parts of plants, matching the specific chemistry to unique biological needs. Ethical businesses which focus on healthcare also seek plants grown in the best geographical environment, with the participation of local farmers and agriculturalists.

When done well, it is an exercise in the *principle of subsidiarity,* and is an approach to health care which honors both the environment (as God's creation and gift to us) and the design of the body. Of course, like any product in the free-market economy, this can be done badly by people who are corrupt and predatory toward consumers. Many companies are peddling synthetic (toxic) or low-quality products. It is up to us to be savvy shoppers and make informed choices. *Caveat emptor!*

God is good. He loves us. He provides for us. He blessed us with amazing, beautiful bodies, the materials of the earth to serve those bodies, and the intelligence to use those materials. That applies to natural, traditional, and modern medicine. They all have a place.

I cannot repeat this often enough—the natural world flows from and belongs to God. He is Master of all creation and, just because pagans use a plant in their rituals or move their bodies in a particular way when they meditate, does not give them ownership over those things. As Christians, we are charged with the care of our bodies and the earth, and it is entirely consistent with our identity to recognize and utilize these gifts.

Recall that the Church herself uses plant oils. At the Chrism Mass on Holy Thursday, our bishops bless them for use throughout the year. The smells fill our sensory memories, carry symbolic significance, and are used as sacramentals. After our babies are baptized, we breathe in the balsam that was touched to them and regret that we ever have to wash it away! Frankincense has long been used in liturgical celebrations and was even given to Our Lord on the occasion of His Nativity by "wise men from the East." This gift was considered at the time to be a medicinal treasure (and symbolic of His divinity). Of course, we do not worship the created rather than the Creator, but neither should we falsely or artificially separate the gift from the Giver.

At the end of day, you don't have to use medicinal plants to be a whole and healthy practicing Catholic. But it is good to know that there is nothing inconsistent about natural health options and a strong life of faith. God's creation is magnificent, and we are closer to understanding His great love for us when we develop a deeper appreciation for His plan for our bodily care.

Your shoots are an orchard of pomegranates with all the choicest fruits, henna with nard, nard and saffron, calamus and cinnamon, with all the trees of frankincense, myrrh and flies, with all chief spices—a garden fountain, a well of living water, and flowing streams from Lebanon.
—Song of Solomon 4:13-15

IS NATURAL HEALTH CARE
SPIRITUALLY DANGEROUS?

But you must not search into the secrets of God beyond those things the
Divine Majesty wills to be revealed for love of those who trust in Him.
— St. Hildegard of Bingen, *Scivias*

---

*T*he question of spiritual danger is appropriate among serious Catholics seeking to know more about natural health care. Confusion and ignorance are common regarding this topic, and there is at least one influential Catholic ministry which has made hapless, broad statements condemning all alternative methods as spiritually dangerous. Some individuals have gone so far as to claim that Catholics have a *moral obligation* to accept the diagnosis and treatment of physicians trained in contemporary western schools and methods (simply because they are the newest and allegedly on the cutting edge of science), and that we must avoid alternative approaches.

There are multiple problems with these claims. The most obvious is that there is nothing in the body of Catholic teaching to support this gratuitous assertion. Another problem is that medicine is always an emerging and evolving science. Even doctors within the same practice or hospital system will disagree over the benefit or harm of particular medications and treatment modalities. It is certainly impossible to speak of "modern medical care" as if it were a homogeneous territory of 'settled science' and perfectly reliable results.

Facts regarding medicinal treatments both old and new:

- There is nothing more or less spiritually dangerous about a synthetic lab-created drug than the oil pressed from a plant.
- There is no modern medical treatment which doesn't have its ultimate origins in the atoms, elements, and compounds found in the created world.
- A rose petal is not spiritually dangerous—nor is the fragrant oil extracted from that rose petal spiritually dangerous.
- It is not more spiritually dangerous to use a non-psychoactive natural substance to manage pain rather than an addictive prescription opiate. Neither are spiritually dangerous when used properly.

Like every area of culture, there is a worldly and anti-Christian spirit which is attempting to dominate the natural health care world. It is as true now that I have frequent contact with alternative health professionals, as it was when I received my Birth and Bereavement Doula Certifications. While pursuing the coursework for these certifications, I found that I was in the minority. I do not embrace New Age beliefs, do not ascribe to a spirituality which bordered on (or crossed the line into) body worship, and I vigorously reject the notion that killing the unborn (abortion) could ever be a spiritually positive event.

It is extremely frustrating to finally find a model of birth support and medical care so closely aligned with the science of biology and chemistry, only to discover that many of the practitioners have rejected Christ, its architect! I have found a similarly disappointing dominance in the world of natural medicine.

Contemporary western medicine is clearly the dominant approach in our society, and the medical-pharmaceutical complex is wealthy and powerful. Add to this a variety of interests (like those with poorly formed theological opinions), and the pressure to employ only what is unilaterally labeled "modern medicine" for your personal health care becomes rather intense. Although the pharmaceutical model seems the path of least resistance, I do not accept the belief that mankind has cracked the code to health and wellness by using medications and surgery as the sole (or even primary) solution. In fact, the statistics (including mortality and disease rates) demonstrate quite the opposite. I have spent the last decade discovering that a more natural model is consistent with a Christian worldview. This is not surprising, because God is the author of the natural world.

Rather than allow negative cultural stereotypes to dictate our health care decisions, we should simply strive after Christ in every area of our lives and a reasonable integrative approach will become clear. *Seek first the kingdom of God, and His righteousness...* (Matt 6:33)

WHAT IS NEW AGE AND WHY SHOULD WE CARE?

At the foundation of New Age beliefs is the fallacy that there is a 'universal energy' which can be tapped into and controlled in order to effect any change we desire—like 'the force' of Star Wars or the 'magic' of Harry Potter. There are many variations of belief about the soul within the New Age world, but they ultimately converge on the point that we have an innate power which originates outside of the natural and spiritual laws of God. These beliefs often combine elements from many different sources. The New Age ends up not as a unified or single religion, but a loosely organized collection of practices and ideas from sources such as Hinduism, pantheism, astrology, Buddhism, humanist psychology, Sufism, Zen, occultism, physics, monism, and even Christianity.

New Age beliefs may appeal to the American spirit of independence because they assert an offer of freedom from the boundaries of religion while still allowing the practitioner to feel "spiritual." They posit, for example, that you can retain a belief in a 'divine power' while also believing oneself to be divine. To the poorly catechized, it may even sound a lot like what they learned in Sunday school. But in Christianity, there is a clear delineation between God and His beloved creation. He breathes life into our souls and we live only through His Divine Will and Power. In fact, were He to cease willing our existence even for a millisecond, we would cease to be. Conversely, it is absurd to think that we could possibly exert control of the power of the Almighty and Everliving God. On the other hand, the practitioners of the New Age claim to use techniques or tools as a magic wand with which to direct and control the universal or "god" energy.

Sacred Scripture and *The Catechism of the Catholic Church* specifically condemn these practices, even when they are in used in the pursuit of healing:

---

§2117 *All practices of magic or sorcery, by which one attempts to tame occult powers, so as to place them at one's service and have a supernatural power over others—even if this were for the sake of restoring their health—are gravely contrary to the virtue of religion.*

The journey into sorcery may start small, with easy mind-management methods (memorization techniques, relaxation methods, yoga positions, etc.) that offer a relief from stress or an easy way to manage or organize your life. However, these apparently innocent beginnings typically ascend up a ladder of increasingly occult practices and demonic influence. I once attended a seminar that began with practical memorization techniques, such as associating names with something interesting about the person. But as the weekend progressed, we gradually moved into techniques which involved meditation and, finally, contacting spirit guides to retrieve 'lost information.'

Another example common among New Age adherents is called *reiki*, which is often advertised as an innocent-sounding "healing touch" class. Students learn to place their hands on (or hovering above) the subject to do elementary 'energy work.' This so-called energy work seeks to balance and restore the vibrations of the body to a healthy state. However, the committed *reiki* student can progress to become a 'master,' whose healing repertoire will include direct interaction with 'spirit guides'—who are really just demons posing as angelic guides or spiritual friends.

Yoga includes a similar progression of spiritual involvement. Most people are unaware that the American practice of *yoga* is simply a watered-down version of the Hindu worship of pagan gods. But, in fact, yoga is one of the traditional schools of devotion for religious adherents of the Hindu religion. Many Americans who attend yoga classes or use yoga exercise videos may see themselves as relatively unaffected by their exposure to this religious practice. Unfortunately, far too many unsuspecting westerners are lured into advancing to a more spiritual practice through increased interest or exposure. This can be a dangerous and slippery slope.

As I mentioned above, "energy work" is a general term for one of the most commonly used New Age practices. "Isn't everything made of energy? And isn't energy made by God? And doesn't he want you to heal?" These are common questions which often confuse well-meaning but ill-prepared Christians. Too often, they are not equipped with the ability to respond with "a reason for their hope"—that is, Jesus Christ—and they find themselves unable to argue with questions designed to confuse and deceive. This may be the beginning of terrible spiritual practices which they did not foresee and begin to embrace. I regularly encounter Catholic moms who have eagerly adopted New Age healing practices introduced by their friends, co-workers, and even physicians. They are engaged in the same activities which I rejected when I left the occult for Christ, but which have been presented with a softer, more scientific veneer.

I am aware that even some practicing Catholics have resorted to using a fringe homeopathic technique called the '*paper remedy.*' In this bizarre practice, the name of a homeopathic remedy is written (in Latin, ostensibly for a more potent effect) on a piece of paper and placed under a glass. The remedy is somehow (magically?) transferred to the water. The patient is supposed to drink the water and thereby receive the remedy. The truth is that these souls have been misled by bad actors (whether corporeal or ethereal), and by their intense desire for an answer—any answer—to their suffering. In doing so, they have separated themselves from authentic science (the laws of nature) *and* the natural law, and placed themselves in opposition to their Eternal Creator.

As a youngster involved in New Age spirituality, I exhausted the library resources, learning how to harness the 'energy' of the universe. In a fashion that has characteristics in common with today's 'paper remedy,' I was instructed that the simple act of writing words on paper would produce a physical outcome (similar to the pagan voodoo belief that sticking pins into a doll will bring harm to the person the doll is supposed to represent). The next step was to burn the paper with the words written on it, to send its energy particles into the universal consciousness. Another common practice is to sleep with words or objects under your pillow, supposedly to direct their energy into your subconscious, so that you can tap into unseen power or receive 'healing vibrations.' Be assured, this is not the same as 'positive thinking' or goal-setting. Rather, its express purpose is to influence and change people and events through the manipulation of so-called "energy."

My involvement in these peculiar activities was fundamentally spiritual, though certainly not in a Christian sense. I was instructed to believe that my destiny was to become a deity, and that such potential was already inside of me—waiting to be freed from the constraints of my physical body (which was only an obstacle to happiness).

My spiritual curiosity and desire eventually worked against me, as I became increasingly frightened by the real manifestations of the demonic in my life. I was reluctant to share these experiences with others who seemed enlightened and positive about their own spirituality, so I did not seek help from anyone. But during the most terrifying moments, I cried out to God, asking Him to rescue me. I now know that He heard every cry and never left my side.

As our cultural ignorance of the Truths of authentic philosophy and theology escalates, 'spiritual healing' techniques fall out of fashion and are more frequently (and inaccurately) identified by scientific-sounding labels such as *'quantum physics.'* On one hand, this is an artful dodge—a simple way to explain a particular faith without acknowledging any references to religion or God. On the other hand, it is also a technique used to avoid applying the scientific method to practices which have no basis in truth, biological or otherwise. The truth is that this type of 'quantum physics' has nothing at all to do with atoms, subatomic particles, or any legitimate propositions within the actual science of physics. Such beliefs includes all so-called 'energy work,' like *reiki, chakras, color therapy*, etc. While it is accurate that a myriad of intangible factors contribute to our feelings of wellbeing and physical health, it certainly not true that every kind of faith-practice is a prudent choice for healing.

It is true that every created living thing has an animating energy (that is, a soul), and each emits some kind of noise within a particular frequency range. It is also clear that we can be impacted positively or negatively by certain frequencies—we have seen numerous studies, for instance, that indicate that there are positive, organizing effects on the brain when listening to the mathematical musical genius of Wolfgang Amadeus Mozart. However, the fact remains that the "energy work" being claimed in the name of natural healing has no rational or measurable relationship with God's design. Rather, these occult practices leave our souls wide open to evil spiritual influences over which we have no real control.

I absolutely believe that God heals outside of the laws of nature. These documented, extraordinary events are known as miracles! Nor am I rejecting the idea that certain aspects of legitimate quantum physics are real and that quantum theory offers some potential explanations regarding the behavior of atoms and subatomic particles. However, much of quantum theory is unproven, perhaps even manifestly unprovable. Experiments with an 'energy' whose intentions and effects are not clearly oriented toward the Truth and Beauty of Jesus Christ and His Church are a significant and intolerable spiritual risk.

In the *Catechism*, we read that:

§159. *There are no discrepancies between true science and faith, for it is God Himself who made the secrets of nature what they are. Since the same God who reveals mysteries and infuses faith has bestowed the light of reason on the human mind, God cannot deny himself, nor can truth ever contradict.*

A key term in the foregoing is "true science," because there are certainly abominations and lies perpetuated in the name of science which do not flow from truth, reason, or love.

As an aromatherapist, I sometimes come across people who want to use the 'energy vibrations' of plant oils to treat people—rather than look to the simple and biologically obvious healing chemistry of the oils as designed by God. This kind of quackery disregards the objective science (which is quite amazing, beautiful, effective, and quantifiable) and, frankly, does real harm to those trying to find natural and effective alternative healthcare solutions.

When I use essential oils or herbs, I do not use them to 'transfer energy' or balance 'chakras.' This is just sorcery by another name. Instead, I recognize that they work biologically and chemically on a cellular level. What a thrilling example of God's magnanimity! This requires no greater faith from me that which I have in elementary science.

God's presence (Grace) sustains the universe and is present in every jot and tittle of creation. And yet, we know that the Divine spark is not some amorphous random bug zapper that we can command as if we are some kind of sorcerer. That Divine Presence is Jesus Christ, communicated through the Design of His created world.

OPENING THE WRONG DOORS

When I was immersed in the New Age culture, I was led to believe that I could control matter, people, health, and even the passage of time with my mind, words, or 'energized objects' (like the paper remedy). I recall being frustrated that I could not figure out how to move a pencil with only my mind. It was a sign of my spiritual failure, and I clung to the hope that I would be more spiritually perfected in my 'next life' (reincarnation being another of the scores of eastern pagan beliefs that are frequently incorporated into New Age teachings). I was also terrified every night of my life for years, tormented by what I now know to be unholy beings trying to drive me toward complete despair. They were nearly successful.

We do not always need to verbalize a concrete 'yes' to the demonic in order to open the door to its evil influence. Ignorant practice of the occult or a reckless pursuit of power over the universe will do just fine. The enemies of God will not shun such an opportunity. They do not say:

Oops! I know you love Jesus and didn't mean to invite me in! I'll just move on until I find a truly malevolent person.

Evil does not follow common rules of courtesy or the basics of charity, but immediately seizes upon any opportunity to pervert goodness and enslave souls. Most of us spend so much time pursuing a life oriented towards virtue that we have difficulty comprehending the horror and aggressiveness of those beings who have given themselves over to evil. They want to destroy God and, because they cannot, they focus on destroying those whom God loves. We need not live in fear but neither should we foolishly ignore their existence and intentions.

I exhort my brothers and sisters in Christ to guard your hearts, minds, and souls fiercely. There is no therapy or technique which is worth muddying the waters of our Faith or relationship with God. With an abundance of identifiable resources for natural healing that are supported by true science and consistent with natural law, there is no justification for delving into such dark territory.

PRINCIPLES OF DISCERNMENT

One of the most common questions I field is, "How do I know when an alternative health practice is dangerous?" In some cases, people want to know whether it is okay to go to the yoga class at the local gym. Others are feeling uncomfortable with a health practitioner but are not sure if their feelings are justified. While I previously discussed some of the common New Age practices, I cannot provide an all-inclusive list of spiritually dangerous alternative medicine practices. Such a detailed approach would fill the pages of this book and more. But the following points of discernment can be helpful when applied to specific situations:

- Avoid methods which rely on 'energy readings' for diagnosis. The methods and results of this 'energy work' cannot be proven or even replicated by the standards of authentic science because the measurements are subjective and may change from one moment to the next. Such practices may also include the use of devices purported to measure the body's ever-changing 'energy frequencies.' These machines are sometimes even programmed ahead of time to match the patient's needs (assessed earlier by an ordinary medical examination). The charlatan then leads the patient into purchasing specific products which the provider happens to sell. The accuracy of these devices has been debunked many times and is not evidence-based medicine.

- Avoid practices which use any form of channeling 'energy' or spirits to gain knowledge or perform healing. This practice is incompatible with Christianity. *Reiki* and *yoga* fall into this category. The practice of magic is condemned by Sacred Scripture and includes (but is not limited to) *horoscopes, astrology, palm reading, ouija boards, seances,* and recourse to *mediums.* These may NOT be used under certain circumstances, or for fun, curiosity, or healing.

- Avoid methods which have no basis in authentic science and are not consistent with natural law, and are therefore an easy entry point for the demonic. This includes *chakras* and *aura scans, meridian testing*, and *quantum biofeedback*. These and other techniques use as their foundation religious beliefs opposed to Christian spirituality.

My experience of both secular and Christian natural healing resources is that an unfortunate majority use or recommend some form of spiritually harmful practices. The need for an orthodox Catholic worldview in this arena is critical. After everything I have written above, you may be tempted to reject natural health care options, period. You may be thinking, 'better safe than sorry,' and avoid potential pitfalls by just steering clear of all natural health options.

But I urge you—*Do not be afraid!*

Plants, minerals, and medicines derived directly from them, are biologically sound methods of treating the body which have been given to us by God from the beginning of creation. They continue to be used in modern medicine and the pharmaceutical industry for the benefit of humanity. Spiritual danger is not inherent in these plant or mineral properties (it should be clear that we are not referring here to such illicit psychoactive drugs as opium or marijuana). Spiritual dangers in the use of plants and plant products are typically introduced by the spiritually questionable actions of the user.

Exercise is fundamentally important and healthy for the human body. Sedentary lifestyles are contrary to our physiology and are a major contributor to disease. Movement of the body is not spiritually dangerous. Any spiritual danger is not in the body or bodily exercise itself, but in the specific spiritual context and intention of the user or facilitator. The practice of *yoga* is rooted in a pagan religion and involves particular bodily movements paired with and oriented toward that spirituality. On the other hand, exercises that are incidentally similar to yoga movements, but that are oriented (physically, mentally, and spiritually) toward Christ can be good and beneficial.

Nutrition is the basis for life, and food itself is necessary and a great gift from God. Recognizing that what we eat feeds the very cells of our body according to God's design eliminates the possibility that eating well for health is spiritually or physically dangerous.

Spiritual danger is not inherent in any of these natural health practices. In fact, it is clear that our obligation as Christians is to actively seek to incorporate natural, God-designed health care wherever possible. It is equally clear that we are obliged to treat our bodies with holy dignity—and this demands that we avoid pharmaceuticals and medications with side effects that may be worse than what we are trying to cure, especially if a safer alternative is available.

If it were true, (as some claim), that natural health care poses an inherent spiritual risk, then I submit that we should never leave our homes again for fear of losing the love of God in everything we breathe and touch! Do not live in this spirit of fear—rather, advance in knowledge of your faith and grow strong physically, mentally, and spiritually. Maintain an active sacramental life, pray always, avoid those things which are obviously contrary to natural law, and become people of such great faith, hope, love, and joy that the demons run when they see you coming!

WHAT ABOUT HEALING THROUGH PRAYER?

There are times when the Lord allows a physical healing directly through His divine power. In *The Catechism of the Catholic Church* (§1508), we read that the Holy Spirit sometimes allows people to have "a special charism of healing so as to make manifest the power of the grace of the risen Lord." But this power is not something that we can just call down at will. The Catechism goes on to say that "even the most intense prayers do not always obtain the healing of all illnesses." The *Catechism* continues:

Thus St. Paul must learn from the Lord that "my grace is sufficient for you, for my power is made perfect in weakness," and that the sufferings to be endured can mean that "in my flesh I complete what is lacking in Christ's afflictions for the sake of his Body, that is, the Church.

The Church has always responded powerfully to the obligation to care for both body and soul with a prevalent and abiding presence oriented toward the care of the sick. Catholic hospitals, hospices, and clinics for the poor are known for their charitable and good works throughout the world. If we could just call down healing miracles at will, there certainly would be no need for these hospitals!

We can show great love to the sick by treating them with gentle dignity, commending them to the Lord in prayer, providing a natural means by which their bodies can heal, and delivering pharmaceutical or surgical intervention when required. Caring for the body does not demonstrate a *lack* of faith, but is precisely an *act* of faith. It recognizes that God has provided a natural (normal) means for healing, even while we invite His presence to console and restore. Eventually, death comes to all, and the decline of the body is valuable final preparation for eternity. Christ is present in a special way in the sick, and in their caregivers, during these times. We ask God for miraculous healing but, at the same time, we work. *Ora et labora!* It is the great work of love to which we are all called.

Although it may be tempting to accept the offer of non-Christian prayer (out of desire for healing or out of kindness), it is imperative to decline the offer of a spiritual practice or modality that is not Christ-centered. And, if a health care provider uses non-Christian spirituality, prayers, or rituals over you or on your behalf, it is best to find a new care provider. The spiritual realm is real—and it is engaged in a battle for your immortal soul.

COMMON QUESTIONS AND OBJECTIONS

*M*ost of us have real obstacles to making healthy changes. As an outspoken advocate of natural health, I've heard (or experienced) them all! Sometimes we lean too heavily on our objections (or even excuses) in the face of hardship. We abandon the effort entirely if we don't have the time, money, or motivation to care for ourselves perfectly. Because I don't want that to happen to you, and as a handy "FAQ" reference, I include this chapter to directly address some common obstacles. Perhaps you truly are at a dead end and cannot make another change. Or perhaps there is an answer here that can help you begin.

SHOULDN'T I JUST ACCEPT MY SUFFERING AND OFFER IT UP? IT FEELS SELFISH TO SPEND SO MUCH TIME ON MYSELF.

Yes, you should accept your suffering and offer it up! You should also seriously examine your obligation to pursue healing if God is calling you to an active state of service. It is an act of selfishness only if it excludes the interests of others and the love of God.

Every single person has sufferings to offer up to our Lord. The question is: "Is this my cross, one that I ought to bear, or is it a cross I can set down by being a better steward of my body?" We can certainly accept crosses (temporary or permanent) with trust and joy, but it is not somehow additionally virtuous to create those crosses by our poor decision-making.

If you do not spend time taking care of yourself now, you will find yourself forced into it later by necessity! Years of neglect will take their toll. I love this quote from the diary of Elisabeth Leseur on the practical application of spirituality to suffering because it helps illuminate the point of balance between two potential extremes:

By austerity I do not mean, of course, anything harmful to the body or to health. I must, on the contrary, watch out for and try to improve my health, since it may be an instrument in the service of God and of souls. But in this illness that I am afflicted with, the precautions I am obliged to take, the discomforts it brings, and the privations it sometimes imposes on me (or at least may in the future impose on me) there is a plentiful source of mortification... To perform these mortifications and sacrifices in a spirit of penance, of reparation to God and to the Heart of Jesus, and to obtain the salvation of sinners.

ISN'T IT VAIN TO FOCUS ON MY BODY?

Fear of vanity is not a good excuse for renouncing a healthy lifestyle! Let's say, for instance, that a woman has gained a lot of weight over many years of pregnancies and selfless service to her family. She knows that if she doesn't manage her weight better, she is at high risk for health problems. She is also unhappy with the way she appears and wants to fit into her nice clothes, look more attractive for her husband, and be a little thinner for her high school reunion.

She is motivated by multiple factors such as authentic love of God, desire to serve others, respect for her own dignity, love of her husband, and, perhaps, a bit of vanity. Our motives are seldom absolutely pure, and sometimes our inclination toward selfishness accompanies our good work and holy desires. However, that is not a good reason to stop taking care of ourselves. We must learn to forge ahead even with our imperfections—and of course we strive for holiness as we turn them over to God with humility, pursuing His will with passion and enthusiasm.

WHAT SHOULD I DO IF MY SPOUSE DOESN'T SUPPORT MY HEALTH GOALS?

Of all the obstacles to healing, this is one of the most difficult. Because of the nature of the sacramental union of husband and wife, the courage and hope of one can be easily destroyed by just a look or word from the other. When you need support to heal, this impediment can seem insurmountable, and can even be the proverbial straw that breaks the camel's back—a devastating blow to the will and to the fundamental hope which every human being needs to thrive.

Illness can drive a deep wedge between spouses, especially when it is chronic. Both parties can feel isolated and misunderstood. The caregiver spouse can become resentful when his or her own needs are unmet and unnoticed. Both spouses can fall into grumbling, striving to be understood and consoled. Grief and loss build, anger and bitterness grow. A spouse who is fully well may not understand what it is like to be sick and can lose respect for the other, wrongly believing the source is laziness or hypochondria.

I am deeply grateful for my supportive husband, but I know many who are navigating this journey alone. There is no quick and easy answer to this question. I would put it into the same category as being married to someone who does not support your faith life or personal growth. There are many Christian books on the topic of how to heal marriages and relationships and I think that would be a good place to begin. I also encourage you to do the following:

- Throw yourself into the merciful arms of Jesus through daily prayer and receive the sacraments frequently. Let Him be your rock in every storm and your consolation in every loneliness.

- Become holy so that your witness of love and joy might change hearts and restore peace through Christ.
- Do not let anger or resentment consume you. It is not only bad for your marriage but also terrible for your health.
- Make healthy changes when you can with a peaceful and humble spirit and not one that is arrogant or inflammatory. Introduce the easiest changes in the most palatable way possible and express yourself in a happy and approachable way. If you are a grumpy or resentful healthy person, your spouse may have negative associations with your changes.
- Prioritize care of your spouse with whatever energy you have. Find a way to date. Rekindle what unites you. Have compassion for the fact that your loss of health has been their loss as well—and let them know that they are lovable and desirable to you.
- Pray for your spouse and for open doors to healing daily. If possible, pray for these things together.
- Continue to make healthy changes with courage and hope even if no one understands. Be not afraid.

IS IT OKAY TO EAT SOME JUNK FOOD?

The short answer is: probably.

Eating junk food is not necessarily a moral or physical problem when we are in good health and our bodies are functioning well. The difficulty arises when a person's poor diet becomes a source of physical and emotional harm. This is a common modern problem in that many foods, which are both addictive and damaging in the short and long term, are contributing to a devastating epidemic of chronic illness.

Is eating that cookie (or the package of cookies) going to throw fuel on the fire of disease and food-addiction? If the answer is yes, you may have more soul-searching to do. Does that mean you need to go to Confession if you eat a cookie? Unlikely—but it does mean that you need to take a hard look at how you are honoring the gift of your body and using (or abusing) your freedom.

Freedom is a complicated concept. You are always free to pass up the cookies in the grocery store. You are also free to buy them and choose not to eat them. But we wouldn't be battling an obesity epidemic if it were that easy. Modern science and psychology both recognize that sugar addiction is a biological fact. So the issue appears to go well beyond whether or not it's "okay" to eat junk food.

It is important to recognize the cycles of eating and self-loathing which are so common. It is also critical to return to a model of eating which honors the design of the body so that splurges are not harmful —and seek a medical, psychological, and spiritual care team that also honors that design and leads to freedom.

My case may be a bit unusual in that it is unambiguous—I have both immediate and long-term harm from eating foods which cause inflammation and damage to my body. It is a gift in some ways to have such a measurable response because there is no gray area. "I want to be able to get out of bed in the morning to take care of my children...so I can't eat that cookie."

Imagine if we made it culturally preferable to fall in love with God's design for our lives! Then we wouldn't need an excuse not to eat all the hidden chocolate at once. We wouldn't be mocked for being "health nuts." We could just live without that emotional and physical bondage and enjoy a splurge when it isn't harmful.

HOW CAN I FIND THE TIME TO BE HEALTHY? I AM BUSY FROM MORNING UNTIL NIGHT, AND SOMETIMES BEYOND.

I believe you! As a homeschooling mom of eight kids, wife, and home business entrepreneur, I have very little extra time and energy. Which also means that I absolutely do not have time to be sick! What if I were to tell you that the neglect of your body over a one-year period would result in a long term debilitating illness? Would you make time to prioritize your health today? Even if it meant saying no to another priority?

I know my answer to that question, and here is the hard, hard truth …

The poor dietary habits of my early life contributed to debilitating chronic illness in the prime years of my motherhood. I would have made changes long ago if I had known the long term cost. It would have saved so much money, heartache, and pain.

How does the average American find time in his or her overloaded schedule? The answer may sound crazy and countercultural.

QUIT STUFF.

- Stop overfilling your life with activities that are unnecessary or trivial. Start to carve out time where you have absolutely no outside obligations so that you can rest and learn to meet your wellness needs. Quit even if it's hard, even if it's confusing, and even if it costs you money.
- If you serve on three church committees, quit two. Or all. If your pastor argues with your decision, give him a copy of this book!
- If your kids are in multiple outside activities, quit some of them and let them learn to rest, too. Get off the crazy train and start to invest in a healthy mind and body.
- Quit social media.
- Quit 'binge-watching' anything, and go to bed.

Time is precious. Quit stuff in order to restore your health—at least until you have your health back and there is room in your life again.

Healthy rest is not found in watching television and eating an extra helping of ice cream. Those are ways to sneak in some temporary comfort in the midst of a stressful life, but beware that they can become habitual and replace healthy habits. They can contribute to a significant or even permanent loss of health, and are more often accompanied by guilt instead of genuine or happy leisure.

If the obligations of your life will genuinely not allow you rest enough to heal, then you will eventually learn by necessity which balls you have to drop in order to survive. It's not manifestly your fault that you are in this situation and it is, without a doubt, a difficult one. It is, in fact, the reality that I am living, and also a driving factor behind this book.

The modern man has more leisure than the men of a century ago, but he knows less what to do with it. — Venerable Fulton Sheen

---

HOW CAN I SUCCEED IF I DON'T HAVE WILL POWER?

You do have the will power. You just haven't exercised it yet! Too many people are frightened off by the notion of inadequate "will power." Such "power," however, is nothing more than making a decision to act rightly and then following through with action. As a Catholic, this is simply another way of speaking about the practice of VIRTUE.

Of course you haven't perfected virtue! You are a work in progress. But to protest that "I don't have enough virtue" is not an acceptable excuse for abandoning the pursuit. You would never accept that as the final word from one of your children or a loved one.

Sorry, Mommy ... I will never be able to clean my room because I do not have any will power.

Nope! Get back in there, kid!

I'm writing this during Lent when the entire Catholic world is flexing its muscle of self-denial. We *do* know how to say no to ourselves, but we too often decide that we would rather be mentally, physically, and spiritually sick than go without pleasure in the short term.

This mighty task of taking back one's health is not the act of climbing a mountain all in one leap, but of hiking it a single step at a time and tethered to a rope called GRACE. I know you can do that— and each step is not just one step closer to victory, but is actually a victory in itself.

I struggle with self-control and virtue, and have found that the practical key to my success is gratitude. You can read more about that non-negotiable element of healing in Chapter 5.

An act of virtue produces in a man mildness, peace, comfort, light, purity, and strength, just as an inordinate appetite brings about torment, fatigue, weariness, blindness, and weakness. Through the practice of one virtue all the virtues grow, and similarly, through an increase of one vice, all the vices and their effects grow. — St. John of the Cross

---

SOMETIMES I FEEL SO AWFUL THAT I LOSE THE WILL TO TRY. I JUST DON'T CARE.

A couple years ago, after several years of keeping my worst autoimmune symptoms under control through diet and lifestyle, I experienced a terrible flare that brought my life to a standstill. The physical burden was intense and the emotional burden equally diffi-cult. I not only had to deal with the disappointment of losing all that I had gained but also suffered through additional losses, including my ability to go outside in the sunshine to play with my kids or mingle after Mass. I lost my ability to exercise, my enjoyment of reading, the consolation of spending time with friends, and the ownership of a creative project which was dear to my heart.

As I faced each loss and spiraled through various levels of grief, I found myself in an almost instant depression. There was nothing I could do about it. On my worst days, when I just lay in bed sick and grieving, I nearly lost my will to live. I did not lose my will to be present to my children or fulfill my vocation as God desired, and I loved my life. I simply felt in those moments that I would not flinch or complain if I knew I was going to slip into death in the next hour. My energy, health, and mental strength had dipped to such a degree that my attachment was gone.

It was an instructive time for me. I had often wondered what I would do if I knew my death was imminent. I assumed I would get all my ducks in a row and spend the final days making memories. The new and strange reality was that I lost the will to do those things. *If I die right now, my works, words, belongings, and family will remain where I left them—because I haven't a whisper of ability to move them before I go.*

I did not die, but the memory reminds me to examine the way that I live when I am well. Is my lamp lighted? Am I prepared? What am I doing to design my life so that when those low moments arrive, I am ready to meet them? It is very important to live an engaged life when you are well!

When you don't have the desire, there are some small things that I encourage you to try in order to be able to take another concrete step towards health:

Pray. If it's just once calling the name of Jesus through tears of despair —just do it. His grace is sufficient and will transform you even when you are unable to respond. His name isn't just another word—it calls out to His very Presence. He will not ignore you. Walk with Him one day at a time.

Ask for prayers. One of the most devout and prayerful women I know (15 rosary decades and Mass daily) told me about a health crisis during which she found herself unable to pray. She was so over-whelmed physically and mentally while she was hospitalized that she was forced to rely on the intercessory prayers of the faithful. It was a hard lesson in humility for a woman who was used to being in control of that aspect of her life. Her message now to others? Ask.

Get help. Put a support system in place (physical, emotional, and spiritual) before you are feeling low so that you are not isolated when it hits. Deep in the middle years of my undiagnosed chronic illness, I cut myself off from active community because I could not keep up and was ashamed. During that time, I found community on the internet and, in spite of the known perils of digital community, I also discovered some of the greatest friendships of my life. Get creative if you need to but do get help.

Give thanks. It is an indispensable aspect of healing. Revisit the section on Gratitude in Chapter 5 for more about this.

Do the next one simple thing that will bring you closer to healing —one baby step—and count it a victory.

ANY TIPS FOR EATING WELL ON THE ROAD?

It is much easier for me to eat well and exercise when I am at home and on a comfortable schedule. A busy agenda full of local events and playing "Mom Taxi" can leave me hungry, exhausted, and tempted toward unhealthy habits. Nobody wants a crabby mom!

Don't expect to find support for a healthy lifestyle while you travel. If we really want and need to make changes, we have to commit to planning ahead and sometimes denying ourselves. Bring food or identify good sources of food (grocery stores, clean food restaurant options). My top two tips for a traveling lifestyle are:

1. Cut sugar out of your diet.
If you stop the cycle of cravings and the cascade of insulin spikes and crashes before you travel, you will be free from the overpowering temptation to buy a candy bar or eat whatever is in front of you. Most people don't realize that their inability to control their will is firmly linked to a physiological process of sugar addiction. Many have never experienced what it is like to walk into a donut shop and be unmoved by temptation. But it is possible. Cutting out sugar and it's accompa-

nying binge/crash cycle will also make my second suggestion possible...

2. Learn how to fast.

This concept is eminently Catholic and also a trending way to interrupt the cycle of overeating and the inflammatory process in the body. It is yet another example of how God's design for our health is reflected in the spiritual practices of the Church! Learning to do without food for a few hours at a time will also be beneficial when no healthy food is available to you.

I do not support extreme forms of fasting nor do I promote a particular program. I am only referring here to being able to go a reasonable period of time without having to eat. By all means, eat when you need to! But also learn to be okay with a grumbling belly once in a while.

SHOULDN'T WE JUST EAT 'ALL THINGS IN MODERATION'?

I once found myself in a standoff with a woman who offered me a cookie. When I politely refused, she angrily insisted that it "just wasn't healthy" not to eat cookies and believed that I must eat "everything in moderation" in order to live a good life. She became irrationally upset with me—but I didn't eat the cookie.

Moderation means different things to different people—it is a subjective notion. Let's take ice cream for example. What is a moderate consumption of ice cream? Here are various definitions:

Me: One scoop every couple of years
Husband: When the mood strikes every few months
Friend: One small scoop three times a week
Neighbor: A giant banana split once a week
Family member: *Whenever the heck I feel like it. YOLO!*
My kids: At every opportunity, even if it causes intestinal distress

"Moderation" in the modern lexicon sounds authoritative until we look more closely and see that the term is often a convenient way to justify our excesses and judge the eating habits of others. We know that it is a movable line, but continue to wield it as an iron sword of truth.

True moderation is the application of virtue and discipline to all areas of our life, but the modern version of moderation is pretty much just "do whatever you want to do and call it moderate." We have replaced "virtue" with "moderation" and our collective health (mind, body, and soul) has suffered as a result.

Sweetheart, you need to have a cookie! Everything in moderation!

Except dirt. Or paint chips. Or glue. That goes without saying really. But when it comes to food, one person's "moderate" is another's kryptonite. It's okay to say no to things that aren't necessary.

If you eat junk food multiple times a week and have migraines, IBS, thyroid issues, fatigue, anxiety, depression, weight gain, and a host of other common plagues, you might want to consider doing something beautiful for yourself and throw 'everything in moderation' out the window. You may just be surprised by a miracle—not the least of which might be that you can say no to that extra ice cream splurge and live to tell about it. The cure for indulgence isn't a generic definition of moderation, it is deliberate application of virtue.

Peter Kreeft, in *Back to Virtue*, writes that "Scripture's cure for gluttony is not dieting but fasting." When we discard the moderation myth, we learn a beautiful secret about ourselves:

- We are capable of self-control.
- Our needs are simpler than we previously thought.
- We will spend less on the unnecessary.
- We can be free from our cravings.
- We can do heroic things even when no one is watching.

If we are Christians, we also learn a beautiful principle of our faith —in any moment, we might be asked to give up everything for Love. Every time we decline that caramel latte and offer it as a sacrifice of praise, we become a bit stronger for the bigger battles, and freer for loving service and eternity.

I'M PREGNANT AND HAVE BEEN TOLD THAT IT'S THE ONE TIME IN LIFE WHEN I CAN EAT WHATEVER I WANT. IS THIS TRUE?

The pregnant body gets hungry! And the body is capable of handling (and healing from) many bad dietary choices. But you should also take care of yourself so that you and your baby can be happy and well.

The rules of physiology still apply to pregnant women and there are still consequences to eating poorly. The mother's health, nutrition, and overall well-being impacts her—and also her baby and future generations. This is not meant to shame mothers who eat dessert while pregnant! This is a book written for people interested in healing and it serves no one to withhold truths about our bodies. If you have underlying health concerns, pregnancy is a wonderful motivation to make changes. If not for self, then for the beautiful little "other" in your care. Circumstances such as *hyperemesis gravidarum* can make optimal nutrition difficult or impossible, but the exception should not dictate the rule.

Food choices that nourish or harm our own cells are going to likewise impact our unborn babies. Attention to that fact doesn't mean that we are limited only to kale and arugula! Only that we should consciously consider what we are feeding our unborn children. Studies that have been done on the cord blood of newborn babies have shown the presence of hundreds of synthetic chemicals,[1] which means that they were brought to the baby through the food, body products, and environment of the mother.

The ideal situation is for a *healthy* mom to take care of that beautiful newborn. It's not just about the baby! You are her number one resource and the center of her whole world. You are also a beloved daughter of God—take care of yourself! Understanding how poor diet leads to inflammation, pain, fatigue, and depression will help you to live with more happiness and freedom. Not all suffering is within your control, but there are some things over which you do have control even in an imperfect situation.

If you don't have the best diet and you feel overwhelmed by the idea of change, don't panic. Just make one positive change today, count it a victory, and be at peace. The world doesn't need more stressed out moms and neither does your baby.

I FEEL GUILTY SPENDING SO MUCH MONEY ON FOOD AND HEALTH CARE WHEN SO MANY GO WITHOUT! HOW CAN I JUSTIFY THIS?

The discussion of affordable health care can become heated among Catholics who value the dignity of all life and who take seriously our mandate to care for the poor. Christians see that good quality medical care is unaffordable for their own families and others, and seek a solution to bridge the gap between cost and need.

What is the answer? Who pays for healthcare? The subject divides us along political lines as the debate between socialism and free market rages on.

In the meantime, you are left to answer the practical questions. Will your insurance cover the visit? Does it have to be pre-approved? Is there a co-pay? What if you don't have insurance? What does medicaid cover? What if you need to stay overnight for more testing? Should we drain our life's savings when a single chemotherapy treatment is $20,000 and I may need 8 cycles or more? We can't afford to be sick! And neither, it seems, can we afford to be well.

We can keep making excuses because of our legitimate or perceived difficulties. Or we can begin to find solutions, one forkful at a time. Yes, it will require a fundamental shift in familial and cultural thinking and behavior. Yes, it is a moral option. Yes, it is worth it.

Medical care is *expensive*. On the other hand, there is hope in the ability of the average family to rethink the definition of health care, so that when we do need "sick care" the burden is more manageable.

Christians are finding it increasingly difficult to effectively provide for the sick and poor when they cannot even pay for their own health care. While the poor family is drawn into a further dependency on government assistance and forced to accept care as determined by some government apparatchik or committee, the middle class family is thrown into deep debt by the bills from a single health crisis. Both end up destitute, sick, and dependent on government social programs. Even if someone favors the idea of socialized medicine, it hardly seems advisable to entrust the care of our family health to the wisdom of a corrupt body of career politicians. It is also raises serious ethical concerns that families should be forced to accede to the demands of a system which acknowledges no god other than itself, has little regard for the dignity of life, and is becoming increasingly hostile to the Judeo-Christian principles upon which western civilization rests.

In spite of what seems an impossible dilemma, we can be proactive in this confusion. We can use the current capitalist system to our advantage to collectively reclaim, downsize, and literally bring home the majority of our health care. As consumers, we drive demand. To effect a change requires that we first answer a most important question: "What *is* health care?" We explore that question in Chapter Three.

BUYING BETTER FOOD JUST FEELS ELITIST. SHOULDN'T I JUST BE CONTENT WITH LESS?

Sometimes, people are interested in social justice to cover up the want of individual justice. —Venerable Fulton J. Sheen

One objection to pursuing a cleaner and more nourishing diet is that purchasing things like organic vegetables is an elitist scam that shuts the wellness door on the poor. I've seen this complaint raised by

Catholic moms with large families, who feel financially cut off from such options.

I believe that the answer lies in getting passionate about learning how to cook at home, eating what is healing and nourishing, avoiding what is harmful, and rejecting an all-or-nothing approach. Rather than rage against circumstances beyond our control, let's give the larger part of our passion to what is within our power to change—and let go of what we cannot have. Perhaps, with intelligent and frugal choices, our own family health care expenses will actually shrink, and those savings can then be redirected toward even more (and higher quality) nourishing food.

My biggest obstacle when considering my family's food budget is learning and working to overcome my ignorance and bad habits. I spent thirty-five years as a thoroughly uneducated eater, consuming convenience foods and manufactured flavors. Now I have to overcome fatigue, practiced vices, and acquired tastes in order to find affordable and healthy options. That generally means planning, preparing, and working more than I want to!

This is—hands down—the most difficult part of this effort. If I won the lottery, I would hire someone knowledgeable in clean eating to shop and prepare meals each week for me. Since I do not have that luxury, I am slogging it out with the rest of the world, trying to do the best I can with limited resources, time, and energy.

Dr. Terry Wahls, a secular pioneer in natural management and reversal of multiple sclerosis and other autoimmune diseases, was once asked in an interview if she felt that dietary healing and natural health care is elitist. Although she is not a Christian, she has a heart for the poor and much experience mentoring them and doctoring them to healing. She answered:

It's not elitist at all. That's just a bunch of hogwash...you don't need to have fancy testing to tell people they need to eat more vegetables. Try 100 days of a grain-free diet and see what happens. People are figuring this out. That's why there's so much information on the internet. That's why all the YouTube channels are successful. That's why these self-help books are successful."[2]

There are abundant resources available online with information on how to afford healthy foods. This is a subject that many talented domestic engineers have down to a science and they are freely sharing their wisdom. I am not one of those moms. My domestic skills are decidedly mediocre, my planning skills a bit shabbier, and my energy level (between chronic illness, homeschooling, and mothering eight) fluctuates between low and abysmal! However, I continue to learn, to grow, and to remain optimistic.

The truth is that healing is accessible to most people if they are willing to start taking some basic steps, regardless of their income level, and in spite of whatever road blocks come up.

If you are considering a change to your diet, it will most likely be incremental as you learn more about what your body needs and how to provide for those needs. It is unlikely to happen in a single day. Start with one small thing and make the change right now.

In the same interview, Dr. Wahls made suggestions about how to pursue good health on a small budget ...

The people I took care of for years were on food stamps. On disability. They had no money...they would go to the farmer's market...and they could figure out how to get a trunkful of food. Sometimes it was organic, sometimes it wasn't. For pennies on the dollar. And many communities here in the Midwest have too much deer. So you could go to the local meat lockers and get venison for free...

When people say it's too expensive, it's elitist; often I see that as an excuse. "I don't want to have to take responsibility for making any effort. I want to continue to say it's not my problem, because I don't have all that money to get those expensive supplements and to get those tests." They don't need the supplements. They don't need the tests. But they do need to eat vegetables.

They do need to learn to cook at home. And you can have very inexpensive vegetables. And you can grow food. You can go to city lots...empty city lots. You can go to the farmer's market and say; what is the best price I could get at the end of the farmer's market for everything you've got left?

I once heard a naturally-minded physician happily admit that this type of dietary approach makes him look like a much better doctor than he is. He makes the recommendations but most of the healing work is done by his patients in their own homes at a relatively low cost.

The pharmaceutical approach to disease often results in an insurmountable financial burden with little hope of healing. For example, the average annual cost of a lupus patient in the medical system is $10,000 - $13,000 and can be significantly more depending on the number and severity of flares and organ involvement.[3] If it's not elitist to spend that amount of money on medication, how can it be elitist for me to spend a few extra dollars on organic vegetables and supplements?

Is it elitist to seek healing? Is being well somehow an injustice to those who are not? Or does wellness grant us a greater ability to live a life of radical service to Christ and others?

For the work of social justice to be authentic and consistent, it must not despise the suffering of those who do not fit the stereotypical image of poverty—it must see Christ in everyone and have His heart for healing all.

OKAY, I WANT TO GIVE THIS A TRY. BUT I STILL DON'T KNOW HOW I'M GOING TO AFFORD IT!

I wrote earlier how a simple blood test identified a nutrient deficiency and allowed me to correct months of severe and disruptive symptoms. It never ceases to amaze me how one small correction (in this case with a $12 bottle of supplements) can make such a life-changing difference in physical and mental health. Imagine the changes possible if we are able to address multiple unmet biological needs? That is the reality of my healing testimony.

Some of your spouses may object to buying broccoli rather than Twinkies—"it's more expensive, and it doesn't even taste good!" I don't have the answer for that problem, but I'm going to borrow a play from financial experts, Larry Burkett and Dave Ramsey, and offer a wise suggestion. If you have followed the recommendations for affordable natural care in this book but still cannot afford fresh foods, quality supplements, plant-based replacements for your toxic medicine cabinet, and time for healthy movement, then the next step might be to stop spending money on extras you don't need. Some people are truly without disposable income, but the majority of us are living a life of relative affluence (sometimes even well beyond our means), taking on debt for luxuries, and struggling with chronic overspending. Additionally, much of our budgets are dedicated to avoidable medical costs.

"Quit" suggestions for those of you are in need of healing, but cannot find room in your budget for good food or necessary care:

- Quit going on a Disney-sized vacation every year.
- Quit overspending at the local box stores.
- Quit draining your bank account on things that have lesser value than good health.
- Quit pouring money into junk food that makes you miserable and unhealthy.
- Quit living like you make more money than you do.

If you hand over your hard-earned money regularly to a physician for care, consider that what you eat is your first line of defense for your health. Unless you believe that, you will never prioritize the expenditure.

I know this is challenging advice and I struggle as well. I look back with contrition on many activities, habits, and things I purchased that had no real value. I am guilty of overspending. Occasionally, I end up selling stuff I wanted in order to buy something that I need—and for a good deal less than the purchase price.

Hesitant? Just try the "Quit" suggestions for a year. Make a budget. Track your spending carefully. You will almost surely find some ways to save. Use the extra time and money to expand your experiences of wholesome living, real food, good rest, and family. After a year, reassess. You may be surprised to find your restored vitality and improved health is a great deal more enjoyable and affordable than your former lifestyle.

If you find that you still cannot afford it, you're in good company. Many families are deeply in debt and simply living like that isn't so. I am not the master over what you spend your money on, but I can ask you to take this to prayer and lay it before the Lord. Recognize that He is the owner of all you have, and that you are merely the steward over what He has entrusted to you. Ask Him for the grace to pursue healing. Ask Him to help push you through that first door. Ask Him to help you give glory to Him through the way that you treat your finances and your body.

Then start to learn, research, scrimp, save, and change the culture in your home and community, one small healthy choice at a time.

STORIES OF HEALING

The Lord has turned all our sunsets into sunrise. — St. Clement

---

One of the most important elements in my healing has been to consciously foster hope and confidence in God's design. Feelings of fear, negativity, and hopelessness easily come alongside illness. But the full truth of Christianity contains the overwhelming and eternally victorious hope of Easter. And the full truth of a lifestyle oriented towards God's design is that some manner of healing is possible. Not only is it possible, but it is certain.

With that truth in mind from the beginning of my journey, I began to seek out and read stories of healing every day. I had already spent countless hours researching the reality and devastation of disease and I wanted to counter that oppressive blanket of information with a tsunami of hope. Regularly reading stories of healing not only brought me that hope but also many practical tools with which to move forward.

This chapter is comprised by healing victories from my community. Each contributor has a different challenge and a unique story, but all have intuitively followed the Sunshine Principle to find renewal in mind, body, and soul:

God has arranged everything in the universe in consideration of everything else, and the greatest potential for healing arrives when we align our behaviors with God's natural, biological, and spiritual laws.

GOD, ME, FOR OTHERS

Fr. Nathan Cromly is a priest of the Community of St. John and founder of Eagle Eye Ministries and the Saint John Institute

As a Catholic priest, I am called to embody a spiritual vocation. My days are spent helping people to live for heaven and to cultivate a life of virtue and deep spirituality. This is why, for many, my journey into understanding the importance of taking care of the body comes as a surprise. But as any person who is dedicated to service can tell you, burnout is real. In fact, I had to face it myself.

As a young brother, I began a ministry to young people called Eagle Eye Ministries. In its first ten years, Eagle Eye expanded to the point where I was spending every moment I could, apart from prayer and obligations to my community, pouring myself out for the good of the young people and their families who were entrusted to my care. This was done through retreats, programs, teaching, spiritual direction, and the constant accompaniment that relational ministry demands. These filled my days with joy and purpose and passion, but also gave me very little time to rest. Over the years this began to take its toll.

I put on a lot of weight. Even though I was young, my blood pressure was high and I became pre-diabetic. In fact, I was compensating for my stress and my need for energy by eating sugar in various forms and pushing my body beyond its limits, with very little sleep and in a high stress environment. I am absolutely sure that this lifestyle did a

lot of good for a lot of people, but I came to understand also that it was not sustainable.

I thought to myself, "Father Nathan, if you were one of those young people whom you were shepherding, what would you tell them?" And I chuckled as I thought to myself that I would tell them to "go to bed and get more sleep." Then why wasn't I doing it myself? This was a question that I knew needed an answer. If I really believed in the truth that I professed for others, then I needed to put it into practice myself.

The opportunity arrived when I was elected as the prior of my community in Laredo, Texas. Anyone who knows me is aware that I have always had a passion for cross-country skiing. Growing up in the Midwest and being an adventurous sort, long escapades in the woods behind my house as a teenager and college student became an exercise that was as good for my body as it was for my spirit. As young brother, a young religious, I also skied whenever I could. It was the perfect stress relief even if I had to do it late at night when I finally had time to myself. What was I going to do now that my new assignment brought me to the Texas-Mexican border? There certainly wasn't any snow there! So, some kind people offered me a parting gift and purchased for me a set of roller skis. This rather new sport is certainly unique. Think of it as cross-country skiing on the black top flat surfaces of the modern day roads in cities. With poles and skis on wheels, the roller skier can imitate the essential motions of skiing wherever he is, even in the hundred-degree heat of Laredo.

I remember one funny story as I roller-skied past a grade school on the border of Mexico. The sun was out in full strength and the grade school children were enjoying recess. Seeing me ski by, one of them ran forward and shouted at the top of his voice. "Hey mister! There's no snow in Laredo!" And his surrounding 40 or 50 companions burst out in laughter, ran towards the fence pointing, laughing, and reminding me just how strange this sport can appear.

But I kept on skiing and, with the help of a team of dedicated volunteers, was able to find health supplements to help my body better cope with the stress that it was under. In addition, I just had to make the simple decision to reorder my vision of the world. If you remember the Gospels, Jesus gives us the commandment to love the Lord our God with all of our heart, and all of our soul, and all of our mind, and all of our strength. And don't forget the commandment that we should love our neighbor as ourselves.

When I read this passage, I often reflect on the way that it is interpreted by so many to mean that we come in third place. That is to say, the order most of us think of in Christianity is: God, others, me. I am third. But when I look at this passage more closely, it seems to me that the actual measure to which I'm called to love my neighbor is a love that I have for myself. If I put my neighbor before myself—concretely speaking—I will never have time to take care of myself. Yet, if I do accept the import of taking care of myself, the misperception of "I am third" can give rise to a sense of wrongdoing, and even leave me feeling vaguely guilty for doing so. Almost as if self care was somehow an inordinate self-indulgence.

Why did Jesus tell us to love our neighbor as ourselves? Upon a more careful reading, it seems to me that the love that we have for our neighbor needs to be an extension of the love we have for ourselves. And therefore, care for our neighbor requires taking care of ourselves.

After all, if I don't love or care for myself, what kind of example am I giving to my neighbor? Wouldn't a love given to our neighbors that doesn't include a genuine esteem and respect for ourselves - including our bodily condition - be inherently contradictory?

How could I tell another person that they are good and worthy of care if I, by my own life and witness, don't take care of myself? I wonder then if our priorities should read:

God, me, for others.

That is to say, that I ensure that I am respecting myself so that I can serve others with the best version of myself. And this care for myself isn't just physical but also implies intellectual, emotional, and spiritual development. That is, to be the best servant of my neighbor,

I need to be as intelligent, well rounded, rested, and creative as I can be.

For me, this meant accepting that the way that I found energy and creativity involved using my body in an athletic way and also demanded having time by myself to ponder and process. Affording myself this apparent luxury actually enabled me to be the servant God was calling me to be to my neighbor. And taking care of my health via supplements and healthy eating has made a world of difference.

I can summarize my experience by saying that I discovered that, if I really loved Christ with all of my heart, and soul and strength, I needed to also love him with my mind. And that means that I had to become intelligent about that love.

Loving God to excess is holiness. But an authentic sense of excess demands that the excess be sustainable and sustained over the whole of a life. If I really love God passionately and with a desire to be consumed by that love in a life of service to others, shouldn't I be intelligent enough to make that gift of service as long-lasting and as fruitful as it can be? Otherwise, won't I in fact be preferring an outwardly heroic display of love to an effective sustainable one? Taking the little way of the saints—the way of humility—requires us to be good stewards of our health and energy And I have found that this little way has also made me a better shepherd of souls.

CARING FOR THE FEMININE:
From the Pill to Crunchy Catholic
Christina Jaloway is a wife, mama, and author at theevangelista.com

As a teenager in the late '90s and early 2000s, I considered myself a "healthy eater" and a healthy person. I played high school volleyball and ate a low fat, low calorie diet. My mom was fully convinced by the health gurus at the time that a diet high in whole grains, low fat dairy, and low calorie, "sugar free" desserts was the ticket to good health. She encouraged us to drink lots of skim milk, eat at least three fruits a day, bought us whole grain cereal (they were part of a well balanced breakfast, after all), gave us fruit snacks (made with real fruit juice, of course) in our lunches, and made sure the ice cream in the freezer was low fat. I know she was simply following conventional wisdom at the time and doing the best she knew how to nourish her family.

In my mind back then, so long as I was "skinny," I was healthy. I didn't know much about my hormones or my fertility apart from the fact that my period came each month, following a week or two of horrible mood swings, anxiety, insomnia, and acne. My mom also suffered from severe PMS, so I figured it was simply hereditary and out of my control. I suffered from a generalized anxiety disorder as well, for which I went to sporadic therapy sessions, but I had no idea that my diet and steady stream of caffeine from all of the diet soda I drank was sabotaging my hormonal balance, and probably contributing to my anxiety and depression.

Thankfully, my mom knew better than to let my gynecologist put me on the pill for my PMS issues, but not even my dad (a physician) knew how much all of the antibiotics my dermatologist prescribed for my "hormonal" acne would damage my gut biome, which I'm guessing also contributed to my anxiety and hormonal issues.

By the time I was in my early twenties, my anxiety, depression, and PMS symptoms were at their apex and I was desperate. I did not have any friends or connections in the world of holistic health (as a doctor's daughter, I grew up with a disease-model of care, convinced that things like chiropractic care and holistic medicine were "quackery"), so I did what I knew to do: I went to my OB/GYN after seeing an ad for a version of the pill that promised to eliminate severe PMS symptoms. I knew, of course, that using contraception within the context of marriage or to mitigate the effects of pre-marital sex was sinful, but I was not planning on using it for either purpose. I was single, chaste, and just wanted to feel like a normal human being. My OB wrote me the prescription and I started taking the Pill.

Immediately, my skin cleared up. I didn't even notice my PMS symptoms anymore, and my "period" was regular for the first time in my life. I had no idea—nor did my doctor tell me—that I wasn't actually having a period while I was on the pill, nor did I know about the myriad of potential negative side effects of hormonal birth control. The relief I experienced seemed nothing short of miraculous, but I also had an underlying uneasiness about taking something that was designed for sinful purposes, especially since I knew that eventually I would have to get off of it when I got married. By the grace of God, I listened to my intuition and got off of the pill after only six months of being on it. I was 25 at the time. To my shock, it took several months for my period to return, which I know now is common following any amount of time on the Pill. After my cycle returned, my old symptoms came back with a vengeance. My acne was worse. My PMS was worse. My anxiety was worse. I was still eating a low fat/high carb diet, exercising regularly, etc, but I felt terrible most of the time.

I had heard about something called polycystic ovary syndrome (PCOS) and thought that maybe that was my issue, so I got an ultrasound at an OB's office. The result was negative for PCOS. Then, I went to an endocrinologist, because I thought that I might have a hormonal imbalance. She took a single blood test on one random day of the month and determined that my hormones were completely fine but that my blood sugar was high. She diagnosed me with hyperglycemia—high blood sugar. While this was only one piece of the puzzle, and I still can't believe that a physician who specializes in hormones would not think to check my levels at various points throughout my cycle, I'm still thankful for the information she gave me, because I needed to get my blood sugar under control.

It was around this time that I discovered Katie Wells' now-famous blog, Wellness Mama. After reading about her diet—a grain-free, Paleo-ish diet that centered around lean protein (from meat) and healthy fats—I decided that I was desperate enough to give it a try. I took a drastic step and eliminated grains, dairy, and refined sugar, which were the main components of my diet. After beginning this way of eating, which is closer to the way human beings were created to eat, I experienced some intense "carb flu," but immediately noticed that I felt better and that my PMS and generalized anxiety were not as terrible.

My hormones, unfortunately, were still not in good shape for all of the reasons mentioned above. I didn't know that the Pill, even if you only take it for a short while, can have long term effects on your nutrient stores, hormonal balance, etc. I didn't know how important sleep was for hormonal balance and, due to my anxiety disorder, good sleep was difficult to come by. I didn't know anything about environmental toxins, or how my personal care products were most likely disrupting my hormones.

The next piece of the puzzle came when I turned thirty and finally decided to start charting using the Sympto-Thermal method of NFP. I did this solely because I wanted to see a NaPRO physician in my area for help with my PMS symptoms and I knew I would have to chart for a few months before they could help me. Sure enough, after a round of blood tests that took place over the course of my entire luteal phase (a term I didn't know until I started charting), I discovered that I had a progesterone deficiency. I started taking prescription progesterone supplements during my luteal phase and noticed a significant improvement in my PMS symptoms. My OB also prescribed a low dose SSRI (anxiety medication), which helped me tremendously in all areas of my life. I hope to one day be able to get off of my SSRI completely, but in the meantime I am thankful for the help in managing my anxiety disorder, to the point where it no longer interferes with my daily life.

Thanks to the knowledge I gained through charting my cycles as a single woman, I was taking progesterone when my husband and I conceived our son Joseph shortly after we married, which very likely contributed to the fact that I was able to sustain the pregnancy during the first trimester, when progesterone levels are crucial for fetal development.

The arrival of my son Joseph, born peacefully at home, set my husband and me on a journey to more holistic living that we are still on today: we've made the switch to toxin-free cleaning products and personal care/beauty products, ditched synthetic fragrances, started diffusing and using essential oils regularly, and got rid of plastic in our kitchen. We try as much as possible to buy organic produce, grass fed and hormone free meat, and use targeted supplements that are well-sourced. We brew our own kombucha, make our own condiments, and try to eat home-cooked meals as much as possible. Instead of a fitness mindset that I used to have, where the most important thing is getting in that 30-45 minute workout in each day, I focus on natural movement, walking, and if I have the time and energy for a more concentrated workout, I'll do one. I'm much more aware of the importance of my circadian rhythms in terms of health and hormone balance, so I try to spend as much time outside as I can with my son each day, and limit my exposure to blue light after sunset so that my sleep is as restful as possible (very important when you share your bed with a 16-month-old baby!).

What this all adds up to is simply a response to an invitation from the Lord to return to a way of life that is closer to what he intended for us, his children. The results of the changes we've made speak for themselves: I've been able to decrease my anxiety medication dosage, I get sick less often (and for shorter lengths of time), have more energy, and sleep better than I have since I was a child. With all of this has come an ability to enter more deeply into prayer, a greater appreciation for the beauty and exquisite complexity of the human body (particularly the female endocrine system), and a profound gratitude for the ability to overcome the biases I once had against "crunchy" ways of living.

DISCIPLINE BRINGS TRUE FREEDOM
Pat Flynn is a Catholic entrepreneur, author, and fitness leader at
chroniclesofstrength.com

Discipline is empowered by passion. Sometimes that passion starts as a negative, and as you improve, it goes into a chrysanthemum or whatever they call it and turns itself into this big, huge, beautiful, and bountiful thing. It becomes gorgeous and worth pursuing. It becomes something you want to chase, rather than something that chases you. But first, yes, most of us find discipline by trying to avoid some ugly and significant, awful, no-good, terrible pain in our lives, so the more we meditate on that pain, the less we stop trying to ignore it or avoid it, and the more passion we have for our pursuit.

I started working out because I hated the way I looked and I hated that everybody was better than me at everything that I wanted to be better than them at. I hated being picked on, pushed around, and picked last for pretty much everything. I didn't feel fondly about any of these things at the time, but I remember them fondly now. They led me into that chrysanthemum. They changed me from a fat and disheveled teenage derelict with a fairly significant dandruff problem to some- body with something to show for myself.

As I started to lose weight, I started to gain confidence. What happens when you gain confidence? Your discipline improves. When you gain confidence, you gain discipline—a different discipline, a discipline that comes from being excited about what you can do, not what you're trying to run away from. The whole thing eventually flips over on itself, like a pancake. And now one side is beautifully firm and brown because you've been cooking it. It's no longer clumpy and amorphous.

All of us must start with a belief that we can, in fact, do something about ourselves and that it's never too late to start. No matter how ragged you feel, no matter how run-down, you're never past the point of rescue.

I'll give you an example. I have a much older friend who was really overweight his entire life—more than fifty years. And in just these last two years he's lost one hundred pounds and his attitude and outlook and everything is just so cool to see. He has confidence now. He's out doing things. He's pursuing goals, learning skills, starting a health business, even. And when I asked why he was able to succeed this time, after starting and stopping so many times before, he said it was because he finally gave himself permission to succeed.

The point of having freedom is not so that you can squander it but so you can make the most of it—and yourself. You're going to have to learn to put off what's easy for what's important. Ultimately you're going to have to learn to impose restrictions and practice habits so you don't abuse the freedom God gave you.

If you continue to gorge on junk food, you're going to wind up fifty pounds overweight—and maybe someday two hundred pounds overweight. How much freedom will you have then? So you should know that freedom is not found in unhealthiness—only oppression is.

*Excerpted with permission from *How to be Better at (Almost) Everything*.

MANAGING CROHN'S DISEASE NATURALLY

Jessica Spiers is a homesteading, homeschooling mother of eight
@threerivershomestead.

I was first diagnosed with the scary and serious diagnosis of Crohn's Disease at the age of twenty-four. I was very sick at the time, so I listened to my doctors when they told me the only course of action was to take several potent medications with many potential side-effects. I asked my doctor if there were other forms of treatment and if diet played a role in the disease and he just laughed me off saying, It doesn't work that way! But deep down I knew that the food I was putting in my body was playing a role in the disease affecting my digestive system.

Over the next two years, I got married and started a family, all the while taking the very expensive drugs that the doctor had prescribed for me. The drugs were not covered by my insurance plan and cost nearly $800 per month, so I had to go to work part-time solely to pay for them, as well as the childcare necessitated by my working. I had been dreaming of being a mother and felt called to stay at home with my children, but there was no possible way to afford the drugs without the additional income.

When my oldest son was six months old, I became extremely sick —the sickest I had been in my life. The stress of having a new baby and being sleep-deprived was too much for my body to handle, so my autoimmune disease was triggered into another flare. I ended up in the hospital, so weak and fatigued that I could barely care for my baby, and severely anemic from the effects of my disease. I had always wanted to nurse my babies for as long as possible but had to wean early to go on another course of drugs that would have tainted my breast milk. Now my disease had not only stolen my time from my baby, but it was also stealing his food. At that point, I knew there had to be a better way. If I would ever be able to have the large family I dreamed of, I could not continue down this path.

God placed several people in my life at that time to slowly introduce me to His plan for my healing. The first was an out-of-state friend who had been successfully treating her autoimmune disease with the help of a chiropractor. In my desperation, I made the drive across state lines to see him. I am so thankful I made that journey, because that chiropractor was the first medical professional to show me what I needed to do to actually heal my body instead of just suppressing the symptoms of my disease. He performed tests that confirmed several food intolerances that had been triggering my symptoms, and helped me set up a plan to begin changing my diet and lifestyle.

The other person God put in my life was the woman who had been watching my son while I was at work. She had a friend whose son was battling Crohn's Disease and they were treating it more holistically. She recommended books and introduced me to the Weston A. Price Foundation's local chapter, where I met people who would provide me with sources for healing foods in our area. Now I had my chiropractor's dietary plan and a way to obtain the recommended foods.

One problem with human nature is that we want instant results, especially when it comes to healing. This is why Western Medicine and medications are so appealing. They fix the little problems quickly without addressing the underlying issues. But it's effective and you feel better. The first thing I learned on my journey to total healing was that it was not going to be a quick fix. You can't undo decades of damage in a few days or weeks or even months. True healing would take years.

Over the next five years, I had three more children and continued on the medications while also implementing the changes necessary to one day wean myself off of the medicine. Five years seems like a long time, but when you need to completely overhaul the way you look at food and the toxins in your environment, it really is not. I had to go from eating a diet full of processed foods to eating only whole foods that I prepared myself at home. I could barely cook rice properly before all of this happened, and now I was learning how to ferment, sprout, and soak foods, as well as how to grow them myself. All the while, I was still working part-time to afford my medicine, and caring for a growing family.

When I was pregnant with my first child, I had read the literature that told me what chemicals and activities to avoid because they could be toxic to my growing baby. I remember thinking that if they were harmful to my baby, they were probably harmful to me even when I was not pregnant, and so I slowly began to remove toxins from my home, mainly in the form of the house cleaners. But part of this life-style overhaul had me also changing the chemicals I was using on my body (soaps, shampoos, etc.), the scents around me in the air (candles, air fresheners, and perfumes), and the places I would spend my time (chlorinated pools). As soon as I began removing these environmental triggers, I began to notice the absence of their effects on my body. You cannot see the damage these things are doing when you are already sick. It takes starting to feel well to recognize the ways they trigger you.

My health was improving though. These dietary and lifestyle changes I was making had kept me flare-free for five years, and my energy levels were higher than they had ever been, despite multiple pregnancies and years of breastfeeding on demand. I was finally starting to feel like maybe I could wean myself off of the medications.

It needed to happen if I was going to be able to homeschool my four children, the oldest of whom was reaching school-age. I spent years crying out to God in prayer to please let me be home with my babies full-time and tried to patiently wait for His timing.

When my oldest son began taking violin lessons, I formed a relationship with his teacher. She opened up to me about how she had been working to heal her son's leaky gut and autism symptoms through the GAPS (Gut and Psychology Syndrome) diet. I watched her son go from completely non-verbal and toe-walking to a communicative, social child in a matter of months on the diet and something in me said to give it a try for my own issues. I read countless stories online about people with autoimmune diseases that had been healed and thought it was worth a try.

After much prayer and consideration, I quit my job, took my last dose of medication, and started the full GAPS diet. It was a complete leap of faith, but I was confident that it was God's plan for my healing. Five years later, I am still on a form of the diet and am medication and symptom-free. I just gave birth to my sixth child, and despite the strains of pregnancy and caring for a newborn have on my body, I am healthier than I ever have been.

The key for me has been the GAPS diet, which excludes grains, sugar, dairy, processed foods, soy, and other foods that would cause inflammation in my digestive tract, which is the home of your immune system. The other key has been listening to my body and knowing when I need rest. I know I cannot be outside in the heat for too long or my immune system will crash and I will start to feel "Crohns-y." I cannot let myself get emotionally overwhelmed and upset or my symptoms will start to creep back into my body. With my body operating from a point of health, it is easier to recognize triggers and problems before they overwhelm my system.

It sounds so easy written out this way, but it is demanding. This level of natural healing is not without its challenges. This is not a diet that I can cheat on or take a break from whenever I want a vacation or to have some fun. I have not eaten a single slice of bread, cake, or pizza in five years. I have not eaten at a restaurant or really eaten anything I have not prepared myself. This is not something I would ever be able to do on my own and with my own willpower, but only by the grace of God. It is His constant reminder that, in order to experience the gift of being home full-time with my children, homeschooling them, and continuing to grow my family, I must sacrifice certain pleasures in life. This diet is the cross I bear, and it really is a small price to pay for the joy of fully experiencing motherhood the way He intended for me.

Western medicine would have us believe that there are one-size-fits-all treatments for different autoimmune diseases, but that is just not accurate. God created us as individuals and our bodies each need different things to obtain healing. Everyone has different environmental and dietary triggers. GAPS worked for me, but perhaps another person needs a plant-based diet for optimal health. The only common denominator in true healing is the fact that we can't do it alone. We need Him not only to show us the path, but to give us the strength to continue down it when our flesh gets weak. Just remember - we can do anything with Him, and true healing is definitely worth the sacrifice.

THE HEALING POWER OF PRAYERFUL EXERCISE

Colleen Scariano is the cofounder of SoulCore, exercise for mind, body, and soul at soulcore.com.

My life and my mission through the SoulCore ministry was born out of devastating personal loss which led me to a deeper devotion to the Blessed Mother. I grew up in a close Irish, Catholic family, the fifth of six children. Tragedy hit our young family when my oldest brother died at the age of 15, after he was struck by lightning.

The death of my brother inflicted a deep wound in all of our hearts and was the catalyst that eventually led my father to alcoholism and my second-oldest brother to drug addiction. The addictions would cause other trials, including financial struggles and the eventual loss of our family home. But, while my dad turned to alcohol, my mom turned to Jesus and Mary and, even amidst our trials, our family home was filled with love, laughter—and the cornerstone was my mom's devout faith. She was a witness of self-giving love, perseverance in adversity and trusting in God's plan. Due in no small part to her years of unwavering faith and prayers, my father & brother would each make miraculous recoveries from their addictions.

Her faith was the spiritual glue that bound our family together in suffering and in joy. So it was utter heartbreak when she died suddenly & unexpectedly. Two months later as we still navigated through grief, another cross was laid upon our family when my father and brother died together in an accident.

In my devastation, the rosary became a source of peace and healing. My devotion to the Blessed Mother deepened in a palpable way. I began praying the rosary while running, and found the combination a beautiful time of prayer integrating body & soul. A friend suggested adding core exercise to my regimen, and the inspiration to incorporate the rosary with core strengthening exercise was conceived.

I shared the inspiration with my friend Deanne Miller, who is also devoted to the Blessed Mother and has a background in fitness instruction. Together we began developing the program and SoulCore was born. Interest in classes grew and beautiful testimony of participant experience multiplied. Encouraged by Immaculee Ilibagiza, we formally launched the movement, released the Joyful Mysteries DVD, and opened our Marian House studio, named in honor of our Blessed Mother and my beautiful mom, Marian.

We now offer youth, college, & adult programs, as well as Soul-Core Discovery Retreats with the mission of launching classes across the country and around the globe. SoulCore is truly an invitation to integrate body & soul in prayer while discovering the beauty of the rosary—a gentle path to grow in virtue and interior peace.

What is broken, God can change to good, but we have to be humble like Mary and ask for help. Then you can heal in body, mind, and soul, and be filled with the light of Christ.

~

YOUR HEALTH IS IN YOUR HANDS:
Managing Cholesterol Without Statins
Bill is a professional speaker and retired businessman

In my mid-to-late 50's, my standard blood test results (cholesterol, glucose, etc.) started edging from normal to a borderline high in several categories. My doctor told me I needed to start taking statins. He even ordered a prescription that I wasn't aware of until a pharmacy called me to say my order was ready! I wondered why he offered no alternatives and also why I needed to go on a lifetime of medication if I was only borderline high. In addition to being the catalyst for my natural health experience, it also highlighted the problem of unnecessary prescriptions and out-of-control health care costs!

My response to the doctor was that I preferred to try dietary adjustments. He disagreed strongly, but that's the path I took. The result of my efforts after a few months was a 50-point reduction in both Total Cholesterol and LDL numbers, well into the normal range. I changed doctors.

How did I reduce my bad cholesterol without statins? Following the advice of Dr. Oz (which I did not mention to my doctor) I gave up processed sugar—which, I soon learned, is an unpopular choice. No desserts. No soft drinks. No flavored yogurt. If sugar came hidden in things like canned goods, restaurant food, whatever, I'd note the amount of sugar but I typically did not worry about it, and natural sugar in fruits was always ok.

For me, going cold turkey was the easiest route. Just say no. Because as soon as I'd start eating a bit of chocolate here, a small piece of birthday cake there, the back-slide was inevitable. Sure enough, after a couple of years of indulging my sweet tooth, my cholesterol-related measures started inching up.

And then, there's glucose.

My approach to reducing glucose measurements was similar to the cholesterol story, but a different path. A couple of years after the cholesterol episode, my wife and I had started sharing gluten-free recipes with my daughter due to related health issues in her family. I learned that eliminating gluten automatically eliminates a huge source of glucose. It's amazing how many wonderful easy-to-prepare dishes there are without using bread or wheat in general. What! No bread!? We even started eating the lettuce-bun alternatives at restaurants— messy but delicious.

That year my blood glucose level dropped from 102 to 82.

No bread meant fewer low-carb foods quickly converting to sugar in my bloodstream. And, though there are lots of gluten-free options in supermarkets nowadays, I have developed the habit of not eating bread. It just seems like an empty-calorie filler to me now. There are a lot of tastier foods to focus on!

Unfortunately, as I mentioned, the sugar habit snuck back into my life. As my numbers gradually worsened over time, I finally told my new doctor I was going to return to a sugarless diet. She is a collaborator and respects my role in my own health care, so did not argue. She said if it did not work this time she would refer me to a nutritionist. Awesome!

But it did work! In the four months between fasting blood tests, my sugar went from a shocking 121 to an even more shocking 89. Cholesterol-related results also declined dramatically, but there's still some work to do to slip them back from a borderline high range to normal. And the good cholesterol (HDL) has risen above 60 (an excellent result) for the first time on record! From my perspective, that's still no reason to go on statins.

There are so many things each of us can do on our own to maintain good health. The first step is to become a health partner with your doctor. Listen to them, and expect them to listen to you. If they don't, perhaps it's time to find a new practitioner!

I think the struggle for doctors is that most people are not willing to make hard choices regarding food or lifestyle habits, so we have inadvertently trained our doctors to abandon the practice of giving good advice.

My biggest takeaway from this experience? Doctors are important (couldn't have done my hernia surgery without him!), but for many things, your health is (can be, should be) in your hands.

Following are some other takeaways I have discovered about controlling my own health without using prescriptions:

My cholesterol-related results are periodically higher than normal, but I reject statins in favor of a dietary approach. At the same time, I don't want to put myself at risk based on a bad gamble. So every couple of years I go to Life Line Screening for an ultrasound of the carotid artery to check for evidence of plaque buildup. So far, so good. But if there was plaque, I would be listening more closely to my doctor about alternatives.

At 66, I don't take any prescriptions, although I do use OTC medications sparingly.

My periodic craving for sweets is handled nicely by either nuts or by the date bars I make using pitted dates and organic unsweetened shredded coconut. Much better than health bars I have found in a store, and nothing bad (like sugar!) sneaks in.

I suffer from "white coat syndrome" so at medical facilities, my blood pressure is very high. At home, using a wrist monitor, results are always below or near the target 120/80. To avoid wasting time focusing on blood pressure with my doctor, I recently bought a digital arm blood pressure monitor to double check my wrist monitor results, and bring one or the other to medical appointments to check accuracy against the doctor's equipment. So far, so good! Hydrate. A summer blood test identified a slightly elevated creatinine level (associated with kidney function). Hmm. It was at first and made me very nervous. I asked my doctor about it. She said, Drink more water. I've been doing just that, and everything is back to normal.

∼

IS SHE NAUGHTY OR SICK?
Caring for the Whole Child
The story of Daisy as told by her mom

At first, we thought she was a very naughty girl. Then, we thought she had a behavioral disorder and possibly a serious mental disability. Finally, we discovered that she was just very, very sick. This is the story of how lifestyle changes completely reversed the majority of her symptoms.

How many kids out there are just like my daughter? How many are being medicated for behavior, masking the symptoms of the real illness rather than being treated for the root cause?

When I consider that question, I know that I have to write our story so that other worried parents can have hope. In many respects, I have regained a child that I seemed to be losing. Her health and behavior declined dramatically for many months and then were just as dramatically reversed. It is a miracle but with a very scientific explanation. This is her story...

My daughter was kindergarten age when the worst of it hit her. The first noticeable symptoms began after a nasty stomach virus but when I think back, I can recognize signs well before then. With autoimmune disease, there is commonly a trigger event—an illness, a period of stress, a medication, etc.—which initiates symptoms. This particular illness (an intestinal virus) swept through our family home quickly, departing after only twelve hours. We lounged around during recovery and laughed at each other as we sipped soup and ate bananas after "the great purge." It took only three or four days for most of us to recover fully. But she did not recover well.

I did some research and learned that her symptoms were an indication of malabsorption which was commonly seen after a stomach virus. No longer concerned, I moved on without another thought. Three weeks later, however, there was still no change. I began to pay more attention to her nutrition and saw improvements through that effort. Again, I felt my concerns alleviated and moved my attention to other things.

Over the next few months, several things began happening with my daughter. Her behaviors changed significantly. I am ashamed to admit that I thought she was simply being a difficult child. Life is busy in a large family and suddenly, she was the needy one. They do take turns, you know!

There were many symptoms which all caregivers of children know can be "normal" from time to time. Perhaps that can help explain to others why it took so long for us to develop a deep concern. Her symptoms included:

Irritability and crying about everything when it was not her nature. For a long time, we thought she was just in a really whiny phase. Our tempers were becoming shorter because of her behaviors. She was loud, irrational, and disruptive. I didn't notice my own increasing irritation until I saw that the short tempers of her siblings. They were like a mirror of my own impatience and I resolved to be more patient and careful.

Her personality changed and while she had always been my happiest, most affectionate, and light-hearted child, she now lacked appropriate emotion with a diminished response to tenderness, frustration, sorrow or joy within the family. She was in her own bubble with little empathy—not even a raised eyebrow over a crying sibling (or mother)—and decreased emotional participation in happy events. Her sensory response seemed broken. In spite of her tendency to cry, she seemed oblivious to actual pain. She went from affectionate to not wanting to be touched.

Her language regressed. She had always been a verbal child but she forgot her letter sounds, and we were unable to continue with her reading lessons. She forgot common words and would replace them with words that did not fit. One example was her use of the word "ballet" to replace having a bowel movement. She would tell me that she was "going to ballet" and I didn't understand her real need, which was to have my help in the bathroom. I thought she just wanted to dance. She not only communicated less frequently but she also was far less responsive, seeming at times to be unable to hear us even when we were next to her.

She seemed to have lost her nighttime bathroom cues and was having accidents in spite of having been potty trained for years. Her appetite disappeared and yet her belly was always distended. Her extreme inability to focus, and what I can only call "amnesia," increased quickly toward the end of this trying period. She could not look me in the eyes and she simply couldn't remember what she did from one second to the next. Years later, she still has limited memories of that period of her life. She also didn't grow much for almost two years. When her friends' teeth started to fall out, hers stayed firmly in place. Little things. But they began to add up.

Before you start thinking what a horrible mother I am, please know that these things increased in severity over a long period of time. There was no dramatic change from one day to the next and some days were better than others, giving us a feeling that things were improving. After raising several kids before her, I knew that many of these symptoms could have been simply disciplinary issues or developmental changes on a healthy day. But almost a year went by and by the end of that period, I was frantically, desperately, tearfully researching again.

Our family doctors didn't find anything physically wrong with her health, so my only thought was that something was developmentally wrong. In every online search, I stumbled across symptoms of autism, and was able to place her at various points on the low end of the spectrum. Every day, I researched for hours. The last thing I wanted to do was to deliver my daughter into the hands of a behavioral specialist without being completely armed with knowledge. I knew that she didn't have some of the key symptoms of autism but she did have a number of related behaviors. There simply was no "right" answer. I kept thinking: *She wasn't always like this. Something has gone wrong.*

Reading about autism, I learned more about dietary recommendations for kids on the spectrum. I also read that there is a high percentage of celiac children who have also been diagnosed with ADHD and autism. The "What is going on with my daughter?" became a "Why am I so stupid? Why didn't I think of this before?" because I knew well from my reading that gluten intolerance is genetic and that, in families with the auto-immune response to the gluten protein, it is common for a percentage of family members to have full blown celiac disease. We are one of those families. I immediately pulled all gluten from her diet. Within two weeks, almost all of her symptoms were GONE.

I can't write or read that last sentence without a lump rising in my throat. My little girl was sinking into a place where I could not reach her. She was changing. Fading. And then she returned. Unless you have been there, I cannot convey to you how that feels. To have my girl look into my eyes and tell me that she loves me. To hug me with strong arms. To take delight in her own life.

In that first month of healing, she walked around as if she had been asleep for years and was just waking up. The world was new and fresh and exciting. She laughed at "new" discoveries. She took an interest in others around her. She climbed up on my lap. She ate ravenously. Her eyes looked into mine. And she saw me.

Within only one month of changing her diet, she began to grow. And grow. And grow. Since then, we have learned that her body was not absorbing nutrients. Her distended belly was a celiac belly, hurting and inflamed and bloated. Her behaviors were not those of a naughty child, but of a very sick child.

Today, she is completely gluten free. She also reacts to other foods that are commonly-known irritants to celiacs, such as dairy and corn; and she reacts very poorly to large amounts of sugar, probably because it is a natural inflammatory and interferes with proper nutrition.

With most diseases and sicknesses there is a spectrum. No child is going to manifest an illness in the same way. While there are certainly going to be normal disciplinary problems with children, I have a growing conviction that, when it comes to very young children, there are far more tired, hungry, lonely, and *sick* children than naughty children. I also believe that there can be a difficult cycle in which frustrated and hurting parents discipline poorly or inappropriately in response to their uncooperative and sick child. Nature, nurture, and ignorance collide and compound injury.

Even though not every child in the family has a gluten reaction, we have eliminated it entirely in order to keep the affected ones safe. The result has been an overall increase of healthy foods. We are a typical family—our kids enjoy their share of sweets, but now we are much more aware. Even if we fall short of our ideal, we know how to correct course when needed.

Despite what some people say, celiacs are not the only people who become legitimately and seriously ill from gluten. Beyond gluten, there are a whole host of dietary ingredients which are not food at all and which we, as a culture, regularly feed our children. Without consequences? Improbable.

Are your kids naughty and poorly behaved? Or are they just sick? Maybe it's a little of both? And isn't it worth a lifestyle change to find out? Do a little internet searching and you will quickly find out that you are not alone, and that my family "miracle" is only one in millions. I give thanks to God for putting specific people and information in my life to help me lead my daughter to health. I offer our story here in case God wants to use it to help you.

∾

SPIRITUAL HEALING:
From Dark Arts to the Light of Christ
Masha Goepel is a Catholic, off-grid homesteading wife and author at yisforhome.com

I'm often told my life is like a fairy tale. Sometimes it is said in dismissal, sometimes in envy, often in delight. But it's true, my life is like a fairy tale—beautiful, wild, full of hidden dangers and unexpected blessings. Like so many fairy tales, it begins in the woods.

Once upon a time, deep in the woods, there lived a man and his wife. They loved each other very much, but they had one great sorrow—they had no children...

For the first few years of our marriage, my husband and I awaited children. I had dreamt of them and felt certain they would come, someday, to brighten the world for us. Until then we waited, hoped, and prayed. We did not pursue conventional medical interventions. Instead, I gathered up herbs and icons and set to work entrusting my lagging body to Christ, the medicines of the earth, and Paraskeva—the old-world saint of home and family. Slowly, our family is expanding. Slowly, I'm learning to find the balance between control and relationship with the natural world: both within me and without.

I'm growing into the wise woman I envision in the last pages of my fairy tale. The wrinkled, babushka-clad grandmother. I'll spend my days tucked away here in my woodland, with a garden full of flowers —I'll know all their names —and a pot of tea on the table.

On Sunday afternoons I'll have visitors after Mass. I'll cut a slice of cake and we'll talk about the little things, the big things, health, and life. I'll listen like an old crow then bustle around in my cupboards. "I have some friends here," I will say "that may help." Off they'll go with small bundles of herbs. Yarrow, burdock, roses, elder.

I'm not there yet, there's so much growing ahead of me, but I'm on my way. Slowly, slowly, I'm learning to trust Christ and this hidden world He's given us. Slowly I'm forgetting my mistakes and replacing them with wisdom.

There are so many ways to heal but I always come back to my garden. Though it feels natural today, finding my way from a conventional, suburban attitude towards wellness was a dark journey. It's hard to know how plants can heal when the outdoor world is made up of nameless trees and well-kept lawns. It seemed there was little there from which to learn.

In such a place where knowledge and connection have been lost, a seeking heart and mind is too easily entangled in darker mysteries instead of learning the God-sparked truth of the leaves and flowers. That is where I found myself entangled. Too many natural resources offer divination advice alongside herbal remedies, or encourage love potions along with skin creams. I learned so much about the old ways of healing with comfrey and yarrow, but I fell head over heels in love with divination as well.

When I was young, I lived right outside the city, in a neighborhood with wide, shading trees and narrow sidewalks. We played in the street on summer days and never looked behind us as we rode our bikes to the church parking lot and home again.

It was an American-dream childhood. Almost. If the brick house with the wide windows hadn't felt so intriguing and mysterious, I might have grown up immersed in the commercialized American dream and never learned to look for more. We were old world, cultural Catholics, perhaps different from what many Americans have seen. The cultural Catholicism of my memories meant Wigilia and Midnight Mass, Oplatek and holy oil, First Communions, superstitions, and interpreting dreams. I loved the wild mystery of the faith as we lived it at home, but never saw the same living fire in our stagnant, suburban parish.

The faith was most alive in the little home rituals. Rituals filled with herbs I couldn't recognize and had to buy. I felt cut off from the culture of my parish faith. At home, the mysteries of the faith delighted us; in contrast, our parish priest downplayed Christ's presence in the Eucharist and filled his homilies with 'Chicken Soup for the Soul' analogies. I wanted it to be something fulfilling and whole and alive, but the church building felt barren.

I learned to look elsewhere for what I craved, digging out dangerous books with recipes involving grave-dirt and mugwort; tarot cards and drops of blood—but they never quite compared to the hidden Christ—the One we toasted on Christmas Eve with white wine and heavy, old-world foods.

Deep in the darkness, I began to realize that the mystery of Catholicism was wilder and more beautiful than my sad, suburban parish had shown me. At the same time, I learned that my forays into the dangerous mysteries offered nothing close to the abundant "magic" of a grace-filled life in Christ.

I burned my dark books, my cards, and my inscribed candles. But my rich culture and heritage of holy mystery? I merely scrubbed them clean until all that was not of Christ was gone and what remained was a shining Icon of God and His wild holy world. Like my daily life, my faith is a fairy-tale because it is full of mystery and sacramental beauty. So much is mystery, and yet also illuminated by the light of truth.

I chose to reside in the woods because it holds a living stillness. I can hear my beloved crows, watch the trees bend and straighten, and dream of the saints in the midst of our birches. My children run down a well-worn path to greet the beavers in the pond. My nights are dark and full of starlight.

My medicine shelf is full of herbal mixtures: teas, tinctures, oils, and salves. I wear a wide apron and cut up fresh vegetables from the garden. I know the earth now in a way I never could have before: I know it's Creator in a deeper and more intimate way. Returning to my faith meant I had to reject a dark, spiritual wilderness—that was almost intoxicatingly attractive—and pursue something deeper. The enemy knows how to superficially imitate the fire of grace, but it is only Christ who creates, sustains, engulfs, restores, and tames the wilds of the earth and soul.

On the feast of the Assumption, which is also called the feast of Our Lady of Herbs, we bring our healing plants to church in bundles for blessing. Then, all throughout the year they're used to heal, pray, and guard. Yarrow is put in teas to drive away sickness, and on wounds to staunch bleeding. Sweet, scented Chamomile is hung over bed posts to encourage peaceful sleep, sipped for anxiety, bathed in for aching skin and bones; its healing chemistry is a beautifully packaged expression of God's passionate love for us.

I've discovered that my Church loves the wild earth more than I do. For two thousand years, in homes and monasteries, the Church has been cultivating my beloved plants. They've known of them and healed with them throughout history. I've found Sts. Hildegard, Fiacre, and Gertrude and learned from these holy healers, patrons of herbalism, what it means to work with the land. Most importantly, I found a place for myself in the Body of Christ.

I'm the little wise woman in training on the outskirts of town. My garden grows green around me, my children play wild in the woods. There is cake on my table, tea on my stove, and peace in my heart. Stop by! The garden gate is open. We can talk about little things like birds and storm clouds, hopes and dreams; or we can talk about Jesus, babies, and fears. I'll send you home with a sachet of herbs and a gentle prayer.

~

LUPUS, LYME, AND HEALING THE ROOT CAUSE
Melody Lyons

Portions of my healing journey are sprinkled throughout this book, but for those interested in a concise overview with a few more particulars, I'm including it here. Many of you share my diagnosis or have experienced similar symptoms without a diagnosis. Whether or not you have an official name for your sufferings is not important. I believe you. If you have symptoms, it is time to give yourself permission to heal.

My life has been a beautiful dream. An amazing gift from God that is beyond even the greatest of my own wishes. Sickness has been a cross throughout but so have hope and joy. I pray that my account of the difficult details never obscures the greater message of the wild and generous heart of the Father ... *He is not a tame Lion!* This is my story, full of details important to healing actions, but flowing throughout with the most beautiful abundance ...

My first memories of chronic pain date back to when I was five years old. The symptom I remember most clearly is the aching in my feet and my legs. It was like a fire that died down every once in a while but was never fully extinguished. That fire burned for the next thirty years, increasing in intensity and spread throughout other areas of my body, interfering with everything in my life from activity to sleep. Every night of my life, I lay down in bed and sank into the inferno. Sometimes it started in my feet, or knees, or hips. Most of the time, it just raged everywhere. My skin often hurt to the touch. My eyes. My stomach. Sometimes, it felt like my very soul.

Through the decades, I experienced additional symptoms (that seemed unrelated at the time) and saw many physicians and specialists. Fatigue. Stomach problems. Respiratory issues. Allergies. Chronic joint injuries. Neuropathy. Endless...

I was an athlete in pain, a daughter in pain, a wife in pain, a mother in pain. And I didn't realize until I was thirty-six years old that it wasn't normal. The first time I lay down in bed (just a few years ago) and didn't feel consumed by the fire of pain was a moment I won't forget.

In my early thirties, I was diagnosed with Eosinophilic Esophagitis, an autoimmune disease in which the body attacks the esophagus. A battery of tests revealed damage and confirmed my account—food wasn't going down and I was in agony. I went to an allergist who put me through almost two years of immunotherapy which, disappointingly, only made me sicker. Prompted by continuing pain that included my joints, I then went to an award-winning rheumatologist. He patted me on the behind, called me "honey," told me I was healthy as a horse, and diagnosed me with "new mom fatigue" (my fourth child was still a baby). Then he sent me an invoice for $600. It was not the first time I cried in frustration over the injustice of spending precious family resources for no return on the investment.

I went to three different pulmonologists over the years and was told that I had asthma and pleurisy and was loaded up with meds. I tried a fourth and was told that I did not have asthma but received no help for the symptoms. I was starting to understand how divided the medical community really is in practice, theory, and skills. Nobody had any real answers for me. They had educated guesses, steroids and pain relievers, maybe a handshake ... and always an invoice, even if they didn't (or couldn't) provide answers.

Eventually, I was unable to eat without esophageal and stomach spasms. I gave up volleyball, could no longer work out . There was no more endorphin rush with exercise; just pain, utter exhaustion, and injury. I fell repeatedly into depression. I assumed that I was just a failure at everything as I watched other moms run energetically from one activity to the next. I thought I was a failure. And now I know that I was just sick.

In desperation, I visited physical therapists, gastroenterologists, general practitioners, orthopedic specialists, allergists, rheumatologists, pulmonologists, podiatrists, and more. I was told I wouldn't be able to run again and left one appointment with a walking boot to help me function through the pain. Sometimes I made appointments and then cancelled them because I couldn't bear the thought of another fruitless quest. I cried over the bills and carried the guilt of using our finances for another worthless diagnosis.

With each pregnancy, things got worse. When I was thirty-five, I miscarried our sixth child and had the hardest pregnancy of my life (my seventh) the following year. Sometimes I felt like I must be dying and that my body was on the verge of simply giving up. I believed that I had an undiagnosed degenerative joint disease (I was right) and I knew that I would become quickly disabled at the rate things were going. I told my husband that I thought I would be in a wheelchair by the time I was forty.

In the Spring of my 36th year, I was curled up on my bed in the middle of a beautiful sunny Saturday. I cried until I couldn't cry anymore and my husband sat next to me and asked me what I wanted to do next. I had no idea. I couldn't imagine what to do next after fifteen years of actively seeking help. The only reasonable option was to return to my allergist and see if she would help me with an elimination diet. A good friend had also been prodding me about nutrition for a while and I started to listen.

My first ornery thought was, "There's no way I'm going to spend more money to help me do something I can do myself." So I put myself on an extreme elimination diet the next day. Cold Turkey. It was a very difficult week to say the least! It was also the beginning of a transformed life.

Within three days, I had full range of motion in my knee joint that I hadn't been able to move freely in twenty years following reconstructive surgery. Within a week, I had dropped a shoe size (correction of edema), slept without pain for the first time in memory (decreased inflammation), and ate with true hunger and no bloated regret.

That was the beginning of an amazing journey of many ups and downs. I had a storm raging in my body and the changes that I made were helping to keep that storm from causing absolute devastation, but the cause of the storm lingered.

A major flare in my symptoms, combined with new disruptive symptoms (neurological, sun sensitivity, butterfly rash, daily flu-like symptoms, facial swelling, arrhythmias, nerve damage, hair loss, anxiety, etc.) and proper testing, eventually led me to a diagnosis of lupus, an autoimmune disease in which the body attacks the organs and body systems. The mainstream medical system told me that lupus was incurable, but a tiny section of the internet told me that wasn't true. So I began a new investigation to discover techniques to resolve the nucleus of the problem. I learned through research that the body doesn't attack itself without some provocation. I had hope that if I could find the cause, I could heal.

My immune system was constantly being triggered by whatever enemy was attaching itself to my healthy cells and causing confusion (this is called molecular mimicry). I knew that if I looked long enough, I would find that enemy, and I did. I went through an expensive (but invaluable) journey through two functional medicine physicians who took me seriously and put all of my symptoms together. Diagnosis? Lyme disease and CIRS (Chronic Inflammatory Response Syndrome). It was not the news that I was hoping for! Even though it was a relief to finally give the enemy a name, Lyme is not an easy enemy to fight. And that is putting it mildly.

I wrestled emotionally with my lupus diagnosis and losses, and now I had another (lyme) with which to contend—and also (paradoxically) with which to make peace. That mental aspect of chronic illness is, I think, often understated. Engaging in an invisible fight for one's life is mentally and physically exhausting. It is embarrassing and exasperating. Identity becomes confused with illness. There isn't a day that goes by when I don't have to acknowledge my unfortunate companion and make conscious choices toward healing.

I wish I could tell you that I have everything under control. The truth is that I am writing this book while I am still on the journey, not at the end of it. I have happy days and woeful days, exhausted days and energetic days. But I give thanks to God for putting me on the path of health through His natural design. I have learned so much about my body and creation. As a consequence, I have developed a deeper reverence for life and for His love for me.

The healing strides that I have made give me so much hope for my future. And hope looks like this...

- I'm not in a wheelchair. Control over systemic inflammation allows me to live an active life.
- I'm not on over-the-counter or prescription medications. I have so far been able to avoid chemo, steroids, immunosuppressants, and other punishing pharmaceuticals common to lupus. If I need them to save my organs and function, I will certainly take them. But lifestyle changes and plant-based medicine alone have given me breathing room and the ability to calm flares (even the scarier ones) while I work on addressing the root cause.
- I can sleep. I know what it is like to live in chronic pain with no relief outside of strong medications. I also now know what it is like to live without chronic severe pain as a result of honoring the design of the body.
- I can eat. I have reversed all symptoms of eosinophilic esophagitis. I am able to eat beautiful, nutritious food—without food-related guilt, sickness, or having to constantly battle the scale. Some people see my restricted diet as a burden, but I see it as freedom. I have learned to love healthy food for what it does for me, how it helps me serve others, and yes, even how it tastes. To borrow a phrase: "Nothing tastes as good as healthy feels."
- I am free from the trap of sugar addiction. This addiction affects most Americans and keeps us feeling unwell and stupid for not being able to resist a cookie. Once I passed through intense withdrawal and cravings, I understood intellectually and physically the true power that junk food

and the food industry have over us ... and the power we *allow* them to have over us.

- After wearing orthotics and expensive support shoes for most of my life, I now wear minimalist shoes and go barefoot without pain.

- I can sit in the sunshine without fear. One of the greatest emotional losses of disease was my inability to tolerate UV light (both indoor and outdoor) without triggering a severe autoimmune flare. The blessing of going to the park or sitting poolside with my children is a victory, which is indescribably sweet. I still have to exercise caution but I am no longer a prisoner.

- I can exercise. For ten years, I experienced a steady loss of endurance and strength with an increase in injury and pain. It was at times a struggle to walk. My joints were swollen. Adrenal fatigue overwhelming. I am now able to run, play volleyball again, and enjoy regular resistance training.

My journey has been about taking back responsibility for my own health instead of just waiting for another loss to strike. I have things to do and people to love. God will take me when it is my time. Until then, I'm going to tell Him "I love you!" every day by taking care of this gift.

FOR THE CAREGIVER

Love is a mutual self-giving which ends in self-recovery."
—*Venerable Fulton Sheen*

---

challenge for the caregiver is that the lifting of another's burden requires remaining healthy oneself. And, in every case, a servant of others is also in some way in need of care and healing. In a caregiving situation, this can involve mountainous challenges, where personal suffering clashes with the needs of another.

The truth is that most people are responsible (at least in part) for someone else. This balance of needs really defines a fundamental tension in the Body of Christ—between an acceptance of suffering united to the Divine Will, and an unwavering dedication to easing the burden of others.

Some of the most difficult years of my life were spent trying to rise to the demands of my beautiful vocation (raising children and loving my husband), while also carrying a burden of undiagnosed illness. As a result of the ongoing fatigue and pain, I became more withdrawn from local community. Instead, I found more accessible support in the online world, where leaving the couch was not required but friendship could be real.

One of those beloved friends is Susan Husband, whose generous heart and joy in her vocation drew me like a magnet. In recent years, our paths took an unexpectedly similar turn when her husband became seriously ill and she lovingly accepted a new dimension to her role as caregiver. I knew at the time that I was sick, but I didn't realize that Steve's story was a glimpse into my own future.

I saw briefly into Susan's world through what she shared—how she cared for her family, managed a household, raised seven sons, and met her own needs. I read between the lines and the sacrificial love I glimpsed was breathtaking. That there were tears, grief, and exhaustion behind her beautiful family photos was inevitable. But the joy of Jesus Christ implanted deeply in the heart of husband and wife, sown into the soil of the family and inevitably harvested for the community, spoke powerfully of Christ's healing presence. That witness gave me hope, greater appreciation for my own husband and family (true lovers and warriors in my life), and has inspired me to keep fighting for healing. When I envisioned a chapter dedicated to caregivers, I knew immediately that Susan's story had to be included.

LIVING AN EXTRAORDINARY LIFE
Susan Husband is a Jesus-loving runner, farm wife, and mama to 7 boys who writes at soulsearchingmamma.com

Man cannot fully find himself, except through a sincere gift of himself.
(Gaudium et Spes, 24)

I first read those big, bold words of Pope Saint John Paul II in 1998 while studying at Franciscan University in Steubenville, Ohio. They resonated in me like thunder. I had never considered my life as a gift to others. In fact, I'm quite certain that, up to that moment, I had lived solely for one person alone—and that was me.

Of course, if you had asked me twenty years ago whether I was a generous person, I would have said yes. My parents instilled in me, and all my siblings, a deep sense of responsibility of caring for and thinking of others. Yet the questions I asked myself on a daily basis, be they superficial or deeply introspective, were filled with "I" and "me," and were undeniably self-centered.

What the great pope and saint was encouraging me to consider in the idea of finding ourselves through a sincere gift of self, was the deep, abiding truth that my life is not my own but a gift from God; and given to me so that, through me, God might reveal Himself to others through the unique and distinct purpose He had designed for my life.

This simple yet profound revelation spun my heart and mind in a fresh direction. It became the compliment to John Paul II's exhortation, "Be not afraid!" Be not afraid to sacrifice. Be not afraid to do the hard things. Be not afraid to suffer. Be not afraid to abandon your life to Christ and to live for Him.

Those words immediately blossomed into action when my husband, Steve, and I were married in 2000. As newlyweds, I soon discovered that there was no shortage of sacrifices to be made for one another. Our commitment to self-gift was stretching both of us in both new and interesting ways - and even more so when we welcomed our first son, Benedict, into the world less than a year after saying, "I do."

Nothing could prepare me for the long, sleepless nights and the constant surrendering of my own desires and needs for those of this little one. The very zealous and passionate "Be not afraid" that I readily shared with others, was beginning to lose its luster, as the daily assent of my will to the Father's was much easier said than done.

Thankfully, there are no limits to the Father's mercy and generosity. He is patient with us! Slowly, over time, as we celebrated anniversaries and welcomed precious new lives, I began to feel as though I was, by God's grace, truly becoming a person who embraced the beauty of self-sacrifice, and embodied it as well in my vocation of both marriage and motherhood.

Our life wasn't perfect by any means. We experienced our fair share of difficulties and disappointments but, despite them all, I loved living the sacrificial nature of my vocation every day. I savored the fruits of the Holy Father's wisdom, including discovery of self through self-gift, that were being made manifest in our ordinary lives. To me it felt extraordinary!

Unfortunately, I had no idea just how fragile my faith really was. No idea that the Lord would take me to a new level of understanding of the reality of self-gift. Life up to this moment was little more than a series of warm-up exercises to ready me for a marathon. A race I wasn't ready for.

Pain and suffering have come into your life, but remember pain, sorrow, suffering are but the kiss of Jesus - a sign that you have come so close to Him that He can kiss you. — St. Mother Teresa of Calcutta

---

The day I came to understand that the trajectory of our family's life was about to change is one I will never, ever forget. It was a typical Saturday morning, the cool fall weather was calling our boys outdoors to play, but not before they devoured the enormous stack of pancakes I'd prepared to fill their rumbling tummies.

As the heart of our home, I've always had a deep desire for our family to share mealtime together—even if it is just breakfast. Several times I called for my husband, but he didn't answer. With five gazes fixed on me, patiently wriggling and waiting for the signal to eat, I surrendered my will to their way and set out in search of their father.

Part of me was startled to find him slumped down on our bathroom floor, his head in his hands crying. Another part of me knew this moment was coming. And here it was. Here we were. Crying together.

The symptoms had begun months ago. At first, it was the occasional neuropathy in his hands and feet. Then, the muscle twitching in his legs. We thought perhaps the symptoms were the result of many strenuous hours of work, but as they progressed in both frequency and discomfort, we considered getting serious about seeking help.

Was it MS? ALS? Autoimmune? Lyme Disease? Days and nights were filled with questions, research, and reading online, but the search for answers did little to quell our fears, or to give us a greater understanding of what exactly Steve's diagnosis could be. After numerous visits to multiple doctors and specialists, Steve was eventually diagnosed with Lyme disease.

As I write this, nearly five years after that unforgettable fall morning, Steve is still fighting the good fight, and moving forward one day at a time with the hope of being fully healed.

When I recall the early months of Steve's diagnosis, I wish I could go back in time and put my arms around my frightened self and whisper into her heart, "Be not afraid! Remember? You are not alone."

Do you need to hear those words as much as I did? As much as I still do?

If I've learned one thing over the past five years, it's that the deep, grinding struggles of life—even the most unexpected ones—are not random events that happen to us. Rather, they happen for us.

I know that's a lot to take in.

Please trust that I'm not suggesting that your pain, or the pain of someone you love, is there to punish. No. I am suggesting that pain has the potential to bring about a real and sincere deepening of our relationship with God the Father, and with others, if we are open to the transforming work of grace within our pain.

More than that, we rejoice in our sufferings, knowing that suffering produces endurance, and endurance produces character, and character produces hope, and hope does not put us to shame, because God's love has been poured into our hearts through the Holy Spirit who has been given to us. (Romans 5:3-5)

To embrace pain and suffering is very countercultural, and very counterintuitive. It is in our nature to resist, to cure, to conquer such things. Who doesn't desire a life of comfort and convenience?

In Fr. Jacque Philippe's book, *Interior Freedom*, he writes, "What really hurts is not so much suffering but the fear of suffering. If welcomed trustingly, peacefully, suffering makes us grow. It matures and trains us, purifies us, teaches us to love unselfishly, makes us poor in heart, humble, gentle, and compassionate toward our neighbor."

It's easy to trust when things are going right in our lives but, when things are going wrong, it becomes more difficult. Yet, it's when we extend ourselves and trust in God, even in the most difficult circumstances, that the more glorious, sanctifying work can be done in us. Diamonds are forged under pressure, are they not?

Suffering takes a great deal of courage. Courage to say, as St. Josemaria Escriva once said:

If God has given me this burden, He will give me the strength!

If God is allowing a particular burden in your life right now, embrace it. I speak from experience when I tell you that there's a special strength and peace that comes from letting go of the life you think you've lost, from loosening the grip on what you believe life should be, and just being present to the here and now.

You may be tempted to resist this perspective, perhaps because it feels like you're giving up. But the opposite is actually true. You're giving more! It takes courage to think and to live this way, because it beckons us to trust. Trust is freeing. In contrast, anger and fear are binding. They keep us from moving forward, upward and outward with hope.

Trust provides the necessary conviction and grace for us to keep moving forward, fighting the good fight, and freely giving of ourselves for the good of others - self gift. The heart that trusts is a heart that is able to experience joy, even in the midst of suffering. Our smiles become, not a facade hiding our pain, fears and frustration, but a sign of our confidence in Jesus Christ and His unfailing love for us.

A very wise priest, by the name of Father Brett Brannen, once said that our circumstances (suffering) can either make us bitter or better. I'll be the first to confess that there are many days when my spirit has been bitter. I've shaken my fist at God. I have pouted and sulked, wept and cried out in anger, because I so desperately want my husband to be healed right now.

I want to be done worrying, done working, done researching, done watching the man I love with my whole life suffer. Done filling in for all the family needs because illness has robbed my help-mate of his health. Done trying to explain why my husband looks fine, but isn't. Done dealing with skepticism, loss of friendships, and even the loss of activities and events we used to so greatly enjoy together but are no longer able to.

Have you felt the same? You are not alone! And it's okay to speak your feelings. This is hard, so very hard.

It is in those searing moments of broken bitterness, moments that are so real, yet so empty and lonely, that I must trust and take comfort in the unchanging, unwavering truth that God loves me. He hears me. He understands me better than I understand myself. And he waits patiently for me to let go of my grip on life, so that He might hold me up in his grace and give me the strength and resolve to keep going.

Choosing to be better rather than bitter requires one key ingredient: trust. Trust is the virtue from which our yes to self-gift flows. Trust gives us the freedom to be at rest in Christ's love in the midst of our trials and our work.

I have found that by resting in His love, I am free to give without hesitation or expectations. It is in this truth that I have experienced peace, when life presses hard upon us, as well as a deep, abiding joy. I am certain that this joy springs from the fountain of grace, wherein we dip our cup of commitment day-by-day. This grace allows us to love and allows for that love to spill over into the lives of others, especially our children.

The Lord Himself goes before you and will be with you; He will never leave you nor forsake you. Do not be afraid, do not be discouraged. (Deuteronomy 31:8)

This chapter, while meant to provide understanding and encouragement to you on a spiritual level, would not be complete without considering the practical side of caring for the caregiver.

Those we love, who suffer day-by-day, minute-by-minute, deserve our deepest compassion and consideration. As caregivers, we awake each morning aspiring to meet the needs of those we care for, all the way to the end of the day. Every moment in between is fashioned around attentiveness to our dear "patient." This is our routine, our way of love, of self-gift.

It took a long time for me to accept that I cannot give what I do not have. The idea of self-care somehow felt selfish. How can I express my own fatigue and frustration when I'm not the one who is sick? My spiritual director was quick to remind me that even our Lord, who is the divine physician, gave his entire self to minister to countless souls, yet wisely withdrew at times to rest, to pray, and to regroup.

If you are struggling with feelings of guilt related to self-care, may I encourage you to let those feelings go? They are not from our Father. Let them go.

Although it's not easy to balance my own health with that of Steve and our family, I have found a few things renewing and restorative:

GRATITUDE: I really believe that one of the fruits of embracing suffering from a Christian perspective is that hardship has the power to reveal—not what you are lacking in life, but what you do have. Little things become big things. Small moments become profound. Ordinary experiences can transform into extraordinary. But only if we choose to look at life through the lens of gratitude.

LAUGHTER: In the beginning of Steve's illness, I felt it necessary to mirror his level of happiness from day to day. If he was happy, I was happy, if he laughed I laughed. While I was trying to be considerate of my husband, I discovered that suppressing my own joys and frustrations was exhausting and insincere. Do not hide your joy or stifle your struggles. Share them with others - even the one you are caring for. They want to be in relationship with you—it cannot be a one-way street of giving.

FRIENDSHIP: I admit that it is difficult to foster authentic friendships as a caretaker. We don't have the freedom to accept spontaneous get-togethers, and inviting others over gives rise to its own set of challenges. But, those individuals who hang in there with you through these difficult days are a true blessing. Make time for them.

SPEAK IT: Even the trusting, virtuous soul needs to speak sometimes. We cannot hold in the hurt all the time! Jesus wept. He shared his heart with friends and family. Give yourself permission to do the same. His strength is made perfect in our weakness.

EAT WELL: Did you just laugh out loud? I get it! Sometimes there's just not enough love left over to feed yourself well. I recently spent three solid months in our kitchen cooking for my husband, who was on the Autoimmune Paleo Diet (AIP). I wanted him to have every bit of nourishment possible, but learning to cook with the exclusion of so many ingredients was a challenge for me! I often had little energy left to feed myself and, as a result, made poor choices. Feeling achy and fatigued, I knew I had to take better care of myself. I could not nourish my family if I didn't sustain myself properly. Take time to care for your body, so that your body can continue to give in the ways your heart desires to give.

EXERCISE: Exercise doesn't need to be laborious or strenuous. Just move. Find that one thing you enjoy and get out and do it. Exercise balances our emotions, helps us manage stress, fights mental fatigue and strengthens our bodies. This makes us not only more efficient in our daily tasks, but also more peaceful interiorly in our approach to them.

SAY YES TO HELP: If people are offering to cook, clean, car-pool, babysit, grocery shop, or mow your lawn—say yes. Let them love you.

This is the body of Christ working together to nurture God's love in the world, and it's a beautiful thing.

TAKE A BREAK: Once a year, I make time to go on a weekend retreat. Doing so often requires that I prepare meals ahead of time for the family and even line up child-care so Steve can rest while I'm gone. All of the preparation is really worth it. Retreats, for me, are incredibly renewing. Is there someone who can help you get a way a few times a year, even if it is just for a day?

LAY DOWN YOUR BURDEN: This is probably the most important. I say this with utmost love and compassion: You are not responsible for your loved one's healing, for their good and bad days, or for their disposition (positive or negative). Please release that burden from your shoulders and let our Lord carry it for you.

Courage, therefore, and with the soul's eye fixed on the goal of eternity, struggle on! — Blessed Fr. Solanus Casey

Caring for Steve through his five-year battle with chronic illness has been a slow unraveling of my heart, and allowing Jesus to knit it back together with stronger threads of trust and confidence in Him. Suffering is hard, yes, but it truly is the only way for us to know Christ to the depths. Suffering gives us the great opportunity to enter into His precious wounds, perhaps to briefly see life and love from His holy and perfect perspective. This perspective becomes clearer as we continue to find ourselves through a sincere gift of self.

Anima Christi Soul of Christ, sanctify me.
Body of Christ, save me.
Blood of Christ, inebriate me.
Water from the side of Christ, wash me.
Passion of Christ, strengthen me.
O Good Jesus, hear me.
Within your wounds hide me.
Permit me not to be separated from you.
From the wicked foe, defend me.
At the hour of my death, call me and bid me come to you
That with your saints I may praise you Forever and ever.
Amen.

~

NOTES

3. WHAT IS NATURAL HEALTH CARE?

1. A.D. Sertillanges, *The Intellectual Life: Its Spirit, Conditions, Methods* (Washington, D.C.: The Catholic University of America Press, 1998), ch. 1, p. 4.
2. Thomas Aquinas, *Summa theologiae*, I-I, Q. 2, a. 3.
3. Sara G. Miller, "1 In 6 Americans Takes a Psychiatric Drug." *(Scientific American,* December 13, 2016).
4. Michael Daniel, "Study Suggests Medical Errors Now Third Leading Cause of Death in the U.S." (Johns Hopkins Medicine, May 3, 2016) Retrieved August 17, 2020, from https://www.hopkinsmedicine.org/news/media/releases/study_suggests_medical_errors_now_third_leading_cause_of_death_in_the_us
5. David Johnson, "America's Infant Mortality Rate Higher Than Other Rich Countries." (*Time*, January 9, 2018).
6. Michael Ollove, "A Shocking Number of U.S. Women Still Die of Childbirth. California Is Doing Something about That." (*The Washington Post*, November 4, 2018).
7. National Center for Chronic Disease Prevention and Health Promotion (Center for Disease Control, August 3, 2020), Retrieved August 17, 2020, from https://www.cdc.gov/chronicdisease/index.htm

4. THE CATHOLIC WAY IS THE NATURAL WAY

1. Joseph Ratzinger and Tarcisio Bertone, *Instruction on Prayers for Healing* (Congregation for the Doctrine of the Faith, September 14, 2000), I, 3.
2. This fact was referenced in May, 2017 on on *PBS NewsHour* by David Eisenberg, adjunct associate professor of nutrition at Harvard T.H. Chan School of Public Health:
   "Today, most medical schools in the United States teach less than 25 hours of nutrition over four years. The fact that less than 20 percent of medical schools have a single required course in nutrition, it's a scandal. It's outrageous. It's obscene..."
   A study done by the National Center for Biotechnology Information further proves Eisenberg's claims.
   Adams, K., Lindell, K., Kohlmeier, M., & Zeisel, S., *Status of nutrition education in medical schools* (National Center for Biotechnology Information, April, 2006).
3. R. H. Bork, *Slouching towards Gomorrah: Modern Liberalism and American Decline* (Harper Perennial, New York, December 16, 2003).
4. David Clayton, *The Way of Beauty: Liturgy, Education, and Inspiration for Family, School and College* (Kettering, OH: Angelico Press, 2015), 87.

NUTRITION

1. R. Mittal, L. Debs, A. Patel, D. Nguyen, K. Patel, G. O'Connor, . . . X. Liu, "Neuro-transmitters: The Critical Modulators Regulating Gut-Brain Axis." (*Journal of Cellular Physiology*, September 2017), *232*(9), 2359-2372, doi:10.1002/jcp.25518

2. Lindsay M. Biga, Sierra Dawson, Amy Harwell, Robin Hawkins, Joel Kaufmann, Mike LeMaster, Philip Matern, Katie Morrison-Graham, Devin Quick, and Jon Runyeon, *Anatomy & Physiology, 1st Edition* (Oregon State University), Retrieved August 17, 2020, from https://open.oregonstate.education/aandp/chapter/23-2-digestive-system-processes-and-regulation/

3. Megan Clapp, Nadia Aurora, Lindsey Herrera, Manisha Bhatia, Emily Wilen, and Sarah Wakefield, "Gut Microbiota's Effect on Mental Health: the Gut-Brain Axis." (*Clinics and Practice*, September 15, 2017), 7(4): 987, https://doi.org/10.4081/cp.2017.987

4. "The Microbiome."(Harvard T.H. Chan School of Public Health: *The Nutrition Source*, May 1, 2020), Retrieved August 17, 2020, from https://www.hsph.harvard.edu/nutritionsource/microbiome/

5. Maral Rahvar and Justin Kerstetter, "Cutaneous Manifestation of Gastrointestinal Disease." (*Journal of Gastrointestinal Oncology*, April, 2016), 7(Suppl 1): S44-S54, doi:10.3978/j.issn.2078-6891.2015.059

6. Mark Hyman, *Food: What the Heck Should I Eat?: The No-Nonsense Guide to Achieving Optimal Weight and Lifelong Health* (New York: Little, Brown and Company, 2018).

7. William Davis, *Wheat Belly: Lose the Wheat, Lose the Weight, and Find Your Path Back to Health* (New York: Rodale, 2019).

8. Qing Yang, "Gain Weight by 'Going Diet?' Artificial Sweeteners and the Neurobiology of Sugar Cravings: Neuroscience 2010."(*Yale Journal of Biology and Medicine*, June, 2010), 83(2): 101-108.ddf

9. Diabetes Basics (Centers for Disease Control and Prevention), Retrieved August 17, 2020, from https://www.cdc.gov/diabetes/basics/diabetes.html

10. Ibid.

11. "Sugary Drinks." (Harvard T.H. Chan School of Public Health: *The Nutrition Source*, May 1, 2020), Retrieved August 17, 2020, from https://www.hsph.harvard.edu/nutritionsource/healthy-drinks/sugary-drinks/

12. Rachel K. Johnson, Alice H. Lichtenstein, Cheryl A.M. Anderson, Jo Ann Carson, Jean-Pierre Després, Frank B. Hu, Penny M. Kris-Etherton, Jennifer J. Otten, Amytis Towfighi, and Judith Wylie-Rosett, "Low-Calorie Sweetened Beverages and Cardiometabolic Health: A Science Advisory From the American Heart Association." (*Circulation*, August 28, 2018), 138 (9), https://doi.org/10.1161/cir.0000000000000569

13. "Butter vs. Margarine." (Harvard Health Publishing: *Healthbeat*), Retrieved August 17, 2020, from https://www.health.harvard.edu/staying-healthy/butter-vs-margarine

MOVEMENT

1. "Risks of Physical Inactivity."(Johns Hopkins Medicine, *Health*), Retrieved August 19, 2020, from https://www.hopkinsmedicine.org/health/conditions-and-diseases/risks-of-physical-inactivity
2. Chase S. Corriea, "Exercise and Arthritis." (American College of Rheumatology Communications and Marketing Committee, June, 2018), Retrieved August 19, 2020, from https://www.rheumatology.org/I-Am-A/Patient-Caregiver/Diseases-Conditions/Living-Well-with-Rheumatic-Disease/Exercise-and-Arthritis.
3. R. Teasell and D. K. Dittmer, "Complications of Immobilization and Bed Rest. Part 2: Other Complications."(*Canadian Family Physician*, June, 1993), 39: 1440-2, 1445-6.

REST

1. Mohd. Razali Salleh, "Life Event, Stress and Illness." (*The Malaysian Journal of Medical Sciences*, October, 2008), 15(4): 9-18.
2. Julia Hogan, *The Psychological Power of Prayer* (Mind and Spirit, June 20, 2017), Retrieved August 19, 2020, from http://mindspirit.com/psychological-power-prayer/
3. Beth Greenwood, *Diet for an Overactive Sympathetic Nervous System* (Livestrong.com), Retrieved August 19, 2020, from https://www.livestrong.com/article/551858-an-overactive-sympathetic-diet/
4. *How to Calm Your Nerves with Food* (Children's Hospital Colorado, Parent Resources), Retrieved August 19, 2020, from https://www.childrenscolorado.org/conditions-and-advice/parenting/parenting-articles/calming-foods/

ENVIRONMENT

1. Sara Goodman, "Tests Find More Than 200 Chemicals in Newborn Umbilical Cord Blood." (*Scientific American*, December 2, 2009).
2. Ben Lynch, *Dirty Genes: A Breakthrough Program to Treat the Root Cause of Illness and Optimize Your Health* (New York, NY: HarperOne, 2018).
3. Robin Berzen, *The Gene Mutation That Affects 40% of People* (Parsley Health Blog, June 1, 2020), Retrieved August 19, 2020, from https://www.parsleyhealth.com/blog/mthfr-mutation/
4. Christine G. Parks and Anneclaire J. De Roos, "Pesticides, Chemical and Industrial Exposures in Relation to Systemic Lupus Erythematosus." (*Lupus*, May, 2014), 23(6): 527-536, doi:10.1177/0961203313511680
5. Amy E. Kalkbrenner, Rebecca J. Schmidt, and Annie C. Penlesky, "Environmental Chemical Exposures and Autism Spectrum Disorders: A Review of the Epidemiological Evidence." (*Current Problems in Pediatric and Adolescent Health Care*, November, 2014), 44(10): 277-318, doi:10.1016/j.cppeds.2014.06.001

7. HEALING THE MIND

1. Alexander Den Heijer, Retrieved August 27, 2020, from https://www.alexander-denheijer.com/quotes

2. Therese of Lisieux, *A Story of a Soul: The Autobiography of Saint Therese of Lisieux* (Washington, DC: Institute of Carmelite Studies, 1996).

3. A significant feature to the heresy that Pelagius promoted was the notion that we can attain salvation through our works - that is, that grace is not necessary for us to be saved.

4. "Total Number of People Taking Psychiatric Drugs in the United States." (Citizens Commission on Human Rights International, February 11, 2020).
   Stats from CCHR International aggregated from IQVia.

5. Aaron Kheriaty, *Dying of Despair* (First Things, August 2017), Retrieved August 19, 2020, from https://www.firstthings.com/article/2017/08/dying-of-despair

8. SPIRITUAL HEALING

1. Suzanne Kane, *The Hidden Benefits of Silence* (Psych Central, July 8, 2018), Retrieved August 19, 2020, from https://psychcentral.com/blog/the-hidden-benefits-of-silence/

2. L. Bernardi, C. Porta, and P. Sleight, "Cardiovascular, Cerebrovascular, and Respiratory Changes Induced by Different Types of Music in Musicians and Non-musicians: the Importance of Silence." (*Heart*, April, 2006), 92(4): 445-452, doi:10.1136/hrt.2005.064600

3. Imke Kirste, Zeina Nicola, Golo Kronenberg, Tara L. Walker, Robert C. Liu, and Gerd Kempermann, "Is Silence Golden? Effects of Auditory Stimuli and Their Absence on Adult Hippocampal Neurogenesis." (*Brain Structure and Function*, December, 2013), doi:10.1007/s00429-013-0679-3.

4. Victoria L. Dunckley, *Reset Your Child's Brain: a Four-Week Plan to End Meltdowns, Raise Grades, and Boost Social Skills by Reversing the Effects of Electronic Screen-Time* (Novato, CA: New World Library, 2015).

10. A CASE FOR PLANT-BASED MEDICINE

1. *Roman Ritual: The Blessings*, "Blessing of Herbs on the Assumption of the Blessed Virgin Mary." (Boonville, New York: Preserving Christian Publications, Inc., 2008), 88-89.

2. William Rawls, *Unlocking Lyme: Myths, Truths, and Practical Solutions for Chronic Lyme Disease* (Cary, NC: FirstDoNoHarm Publishing, 2017).

3. Qing Liu, Xiao Meng, Ya Li, Cai-Ning Zhao, Guo-Yi Tang, and Hua-Bin Li, "Antibacterial and Antifungal Activities of Spices." (*International Journal of Molecular Sciences*, June, 2017), 18(6): 1283, doi:10.3390/ijms18061283

4. Simon Kirste, Markus Treier, Sabine Jolie Wehrle, Gerhild Becker, Mona Abdel-Tawab, Kathleen Gerbeth, Martin Johannes Hug, Beate Lubrich, Anca-Ligia Grosu, and Felix Momm, "Boswellia Serrata Acts on Cerebral Edema in Patients Irradiated

for Brain Tumors: a Prospective, Randomized, Placebo-controlled, Double-blind Pilot Trial." (*Cancer*, August 15, 2011), 117(16): 3788-95, doi:10.1002/cncr.25945

5. Noura S. Dosoky and William N. Setzer, "Biological Activities and Safety of *Citrus* spp. Essential Oils." (*International Journal of Molecular Sciences*, July, 2018), 19(7): 1966, doi:10.3390/ijms19071966

6. Abbas Meamarbashi, "Instant Effects of Peppermint Essential Oil on the Physiological Parameters and Exercise Performance." (*Avicenna Journal of Phytomedicine*, Jan-Feb, 2014), 4(1): 72-78.

12. COMMON QUESTIONS AND OBJECTIONS

1. Sara Goodman, "Tests Find More Than 200 Chemicals in Newborn Umbilical Cord Blood." (*Scientific American*. December 2, 2009), Retrieved September 8, 2020, from https://www.scientificamerican.com/article/newborn-babies-chemicals-exposure-bpa/

2. Angie Alt, "Real Food on a Budget w/ Terry Wahls." (Autoimmune Wellness, April 2, 2018), Retrieved September 8, 2020, from https://autoimmunewellness.com/s3-e1-real-food-budget-w-terry-wahls/

3. "How Much Does Lupus Treatment Cost?" (CostHelper Health), Retrieved September 8, 2020, from healthhttps://health.costhelper.com/lupus-treatment-cost.html

ACKNOWLEDGMENTS

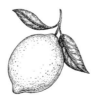

The first fruits of my gratitude go to Jesus Christ: Author of my dream; Lover of my Soul.

I am also grateful to Christopher, without whom I would probably still be wandering around a rugby field somewhere. For this amazing life and our nine precious children. For safeguarding the space around our family and home so that we can live with peace and joy. For showing me my worth, giving me the space to write, and for being an extraordinary editor.

Our incredible kids—for your sacrifices and joyful support which have allowed me to heal and to write.

My parents (by blood and marriage)—for all that you have done to help me grow into the beautiful life God ordained for me.

My spiritual Fathers—you have restored me many times through your wisdom and the sacraments. You have taught me faithfulness through the witness of your lives.

My health care team and especially my physicians who have looked me in the eyes and said "I believe you" and "There is hope."

To the contributors of this book—for offering your testimony of hope and healing. May your words start a ripple effect of joy through generations.

To all those in my local and online communities who have loved me, challenged me, taught me, upheld me, corrected me, encouraged me, and inspired me. I can't list you all but I thank you sincerely for your yes to love.

Made in the USA
Coppell, TX
08 February 2021